A fragile hold

ALSO BY RUTH COTTON

Reinventing Success:
Find Happiness, Satisfaction and Balance
by Managing Change in Your Life,
Random House Australia, 1996

Hidden Hamilton:
Uncovering Stories of Hamilton, NSW,
Hunter Press, Newcastle, 2014

More Hidden Hamilton:
Further Stories of People, Place
and Community,
Hunter Press, Newcastle, 2016

On Wahroonga:
An Early Settler Family at
Rocky Creek, NSW,
Ruth Cotton, Australia, 2017

A FRAGILE HOLD

Living with multiple sclerosis
and other uncertainties

Ruth Cotton

LIGHTLEAF PRESS

First published 2023 by Lightleaf Press
PO BOX 269
Hamilton NSW 2303
Email: lightleaf95@gmail.com

© Ruth Cotton 2023

All rights reserved. No part of this book may be reproduced, copied, scanned, stored in a retrieval system, recorded, or transmitted, in any form or by any means, without prior permission in writing from the publisher. The *Copyright Act 1968* permits a maximum of one chapter, or 10 per cent of this book, whichever is the greater, to be photocopied by an educational institution for educational purposes, provided the institution (or the body that administers it) has given a remuneration notice to the Copyright Agency (Australia) under Copyright Act.

A catalogue record for this book is available from the National Library of Australia.

ISBN 978-0-6481286-1-8 (paperback)
ISBN 978-0-6481286-2-5 (epub)

Edited by Shelley Kenigsberg
Design/Illustration by Andy Bridge
Typeset by Sarah Lahay
Proofreading by Susan McCreery
Printed and bound by Lightning Source

Contents

Prologue	vii
Chapter 1: Lie of the Land	1
Chapter 2: Flux	33
Chapter 3: Shedding Skins	61
Chapter 4: Tracks in the Sand	89
Chapter 5: Befriending the Brain	121
Chapter 6: Sifting	149
Chapter 7: Things Fall Apart	181
Chapter 8: Acts of Possession	215
Chapter 9: Better than Expected	245
Chapter 10: In Focus	267
Acknowledgements	303
Permissions	305
Bibliography	311
About Ruth Cotton	315

PROLOGUE

Once, I was strong. A young woman, who rode horses, mustered sheep, and competed in show jumping. Carried her toddlers with ease, helped set up the tent on camping holidays. That's physical strength. I've always had the mental kind — an inner confidence and sureness that seemed convincing, from the outside. It is with me today, softened by life.

Now, in my seventh decade, salute to the sun in my yoga practice is as far beyond me as springing into the saddle. And hauling myself up from the floor is mortifying.

I was in my early 50s in 1997 when the diagnosis was confirmed: multiple sclerosis.

Leaving the neurologist's rooms, I found my way back to my car along a suburban street. In one hour, my world had changed, forever. As I passed each front garden, bright and still in the autumn sunshine, I remember seeing the edges of each flower and leaf limned with light.

As the years passed, the disease stayed close. I called it my watchdog. Step out of line, and it barks. Stress, overdoing it and heat were the main offenders.

I continued to work for 15 years until my retirement, enjoying a full life. Having my own business gave me control over timelines and commitments, but I still drove myself relentlessly. Periods of high-intensity work and travel often ended in collapse from exhaustion. Stress exacts its price.

Eight years ago I could walk a kilometre to the Hamilton railway station and back again, with a couple of brief rests. I could stand unsupported in front of a crowd at the launch of one of my books and speak for 10 minutes. Now I walk nowhere without an aid; 1000 paces with a walker represents my personal best. When I relinquished my drivers licence, I became dependent on my husband and others for transport. I've changed my dentist because I could no longer get up the stairs to his surgery.

Fortitude is part of my heritage. My grandfather was one of Australia's pioneer settlers. I remember the clasp of his workman's hands, so large and muscular, formed by a lifetime wresting productive land for sheep and crops from the grasp of forest and scrub. When a hurtling sheep knocked him over in the yards, he broke his hip and never walked independently again.

My grandfather, whom we called Dar, was in his early 80s then. Each morning after breakfast, my father would help him down the back steps of our homestead and settle him in a cane chair. I was about seven and, sliding past my father's legs, I'd quickly take up my position at Dar's side. As the hours passed, we'd tell each other stories, or simply sit, bound in stillness. It was of no consequence that he was old, or immobile — he was there for me. Dar continued to be my anchor, and when I left home to attend boarding school, he was a faithful correspondent. How I seized upon those letters, addressed to me in his trembling hand.

Now I have grandchildren of my own. I love how unselfconscious they are, chattering as we cross the street, me walking funny. They don't care how we look.

Once, I was a strong young woman, with a confident stride. My losses mount. Yet they connect me to a world of losses. I know how it feels, to be one of those who have lost something, or someone. And I see that youth is no protection.

It doesn't matter, my walking — or not walking. I hold onto my grandfather, to what he left me. The knowing that staying still, being present for someone, is a gift.

This is my life.

CHAPTER ONE

Lie of the Land

Shaken

I returned to writing after a three-year break because I felt my days were filled with activities that gave me a sense of control over many things that didn't matter, but none over the unknowns looming just beyond my sight. And while completing small tasks yielded transient satisfaction, the pleasure I usually found in daily life had fled.

When a friend and former colleague, David Lowe, emailed from Bangkok suggesting I watch the highlights of the New York Metropolitan Opera's *At Home Gala Concert*, I was feeling distracted and overwrought. I was not in the mood to relax in front of the computer and explore the MetOpera website. Yet I understood that David wanted me to share in a musical experience that would transport me far from the everyday, boost my spirits, bring me joy. I replied to him with a prevaricating excuse.

Why was I feeling like this? My husband, Ken, had been diagnosed with malignant melanoma in 2009. Years later, as it progressed slowly, he reached Stage 4, the most advanced stage. The cancer had metastasised from its original site on his back to distant organs in his body.

When it was found in his lungs and his doctors agreed to 'watch and wait', I accepted that I'd be devoting much of 2020 to Ken's care and support. The year would be unpredictable; I'd be unwise to embark on a single large project like a new book that may be often interrupted. In a New Year's resolution, I set a goal of writing one micro-essay a month, as if I was attending a writers group. I wrote my first, honed it well, then set it aside. No more followed. There I was then, five months later, feeling that unless I started writing again, I'd lose myself. Opera was no solace.

So it was that in addition to my multiple sclerosis (MS), Ken's cancer became a large uncertainty in my life. There was another. During February, word began to surface of a new virus in China, a coronavirus that had jumped species, possibly from bats to humans. Working with my grandson Cassius (Cass) on a public-speaking project for school, we skimmed possible topics on the internet. One appealed to him: *People should be very careful about eating wild animals.* Together we researched the wild animal markets in China, the way animals were trapped and held in captivity and sold; and the thousands of people already infected with the coronavirus. Memory prompt cards were prepared; he practised with his speech therapist to pronounce 'coronavirus' perfectly and, in time, presented his talk to the class.

Few of us realised how radically this virus would change our known world. Later, as schools closed, his dad lost his job, and social distancing forbade visits and hugs with grandparents like us, I wondered if eight-year-old Cass might have felt he was somehow responsible for this catastrophe. In all our conversations though, there was no sign it worried him.

Throughout March, preoccupation with national responses to the epidemic, soon to be declared a pandemic, took over our lives. We came to understand that COVID-19 was the disease caused by a new coronavirus called SARS-CoV-2. Daily press briefings by chief health officers and politicians dominated our media; so, too, the mesmerising stream of statistics — cases testing positive, deaths, recoveries. My gym and library closed promptly; local stores insisted on delivering groceries and pharmacy items to vulnerable customers like me. We were not wanted in-store: I was almost waved out of one pharmacy until rescued by the owner. Months lay ahead of being confined indoors, banned from the social activities that kept us connected to family, friends and our wider culture.

As retirees, Ken and I were fortunate in that our income was secure. But we were concerned about our children and their families. How could parents manage home schooling while working from home? If parents became infected, who would care for the grandchildren, since we elders were off limits?

In the midst of these practical considerations, I knew my own wellbeing could be at risk. I turned for sustenance to a remembered classic from the 1990s, *The Artist's Way* by American writer Julia Cameron. Her vocation is freeing people's creativity, whether painter, dancer, writer, filmmaker or lawyer; her specialty is removing blocks to whatever creative endeavour a person seeks. I was attracted to one of her key tools for a writer's creative recovery: the morning pages.

The idea is simple: she exhorts her readers to write, by hand, three pages every morning without fail. Write, she says, whatever comes to mind. No censoring, no editing. Just write, no matter how mundane. To be creative, one must find one's creativity — and morning pages are the means to uncover and release it.

I'd followed Julia Cameron's pathway in the 1990s, alongside writing my first published book. Nearly three decades later I adapted her method to suit my purpose. My stationery cupboard was stacked with journals written across 30 years, but I'd ceased this practice. I was drawn back to my New Year's resolve to write a micro-essay each month, the distillation of a moment, a memory, or some element of my experience that helped shape my identity.

In a further adaptation, I'd write two, maybe three or four a month, less than 1000 words, preferably shorter. That was doable. Longhand as recommended by Cameron was gone; I'd use my computer. And I'd publish my offerings in a private blog, shared with a small number of invited friends and fellow writers — my own online writers group. I couldn't control the outcomes of my life, but I could influence them.

This, I believed, was the way I would rediscover joy.

Undaunted

'**Without medication you'll** be bedridden within five years,' the neurologist declared, holding me in her gaze. 'I'm not sure how you've managed to do so well all this time, with no MS drugs.'

After the initial shock, I rallied to my defence. 'I did try Gilenya in 2011,' I said, 'soon after it came out. But it devastated my white blood cell count. I chose not to put myself at constant risk of infections. I wanted to be able to spend time with my grandkids — and they always have colds!'

Dr S's face softened. 'Of course,' she acknowledged. 'But now you can try something different. Tecfidera.'

Ken and I had moved to Newcastle in 2012, having spent almost nine years on the far north coast. I think Dr S surmised I'd put my trust in complementary therapies, but this wasn't so. I'd continued to see my North Sydney neurologist and monitor my health status. Prior to his suggesting Gilenya, there had been no bespoke oral treatments for MS, only self-injection, or infusions into the bloodstream delivered in an outpatient setting. Over that time I'd managed with short courses of corticosteroid tablets when exacerbations struck me.

It was 2015 when we were having this discussion, and I'd joined the hundreds of people with MS around the region who were drawn to the MS Clinic at John Hunter Hospital in Newcastle. Dr S has dedicated herself to research and clinical care that will improve the lives of people with MS. One aspect of the disease she seeks to influence is minimising the chances of a person with MS ending up in a wheelchair. She is lively and good-humoured. I've always liked and respected her.

But in that first consultation, her bald statement predicting I would be bedridden in five years shocked and dismayed me. Around 80 per cent of people with MS experience difficulties walking within 10–15 years of their diagnosis. I'd been noticing over some years that the distance I was able to walk without rests was becoming shorter. In late 2014 I had bought a mobility scooter so I could get to the shops and back without becoming exhausted. Using my cane, I was able to enter the shops and collect what I needed. Later, when it became difficult to stay upright holding both a shopping basket and my cane, I progressed to carrying a light walker on the back of my scooter to take into the shops.

The advent of disease-modifying therapies (DMTs) such as Gilenya, taken as a tablet, was a game-changer. I did try Tecfidera as Dr S recommended but the adverse impact on my white blood cell count was even greater than Gilenya. Dr S counselled me to stop taking it. No other DMT can help me. I fall in the category she first put me in, a person with MS who has not had sustained treatment with a DMT.

Five years have passed since her prediction; my mobility is impaired, but I am not in a wheelchair, and I am certainly not bedridden.

That said, I am at risk of falls; I have severe degenerative disease in my lumbar spine and a very weak right leg with foot drop. I wear a brace all day to prevent my foot from scraping the ground. Should I fall and fracture or break my hip, the consequences for my future care could be dire.

In the late 1980s, long before I was diagnosed with MS, I dreamed I was in a wheelchair. I was travelling overseas and exploring a site of some Roman ruins. I don't recall if anyone was with me. Beyond the site was a busy shopping esplanade and then the sea, flat and grey. The site itself was strewn with fallen columns and other debris. I wheeled up to a column that was blocking my way, rose from the wheelchair and lifted it over the obstacle. Stabilising myself by holding the chair, I clambered over the column and and sat down again.

Awake, I was puzzled. How could I be needing a wheelchair yet still able to walk at least a bit? Wasn't I a fake?

The dream was prescient, as this is exactly my situation today — only I am not a fake. As I step off my mobility scooter and lift my walker off the back to enter a shop, I feel pleased with my independence. I can still walk but not far. Occasionally people stop and tell me what a great idea it is to carry a walker on my scooter. I am following the example of a local friend, Jan, who also has MS.

'I agree,' I reply. 'It's far better than crashing into the grocery shelves at any minute!'

Who knows, I might end up in a wheelchair — or even like my brother, John, who has Parkinson's disease and is unable to get out of bed. These days my efforts are directed at managing my disability, with Ken's support and mechanical ingenuity. Without the protection of an MS drug, my focus is on keeping physically strong, picking up new ideas, trying different aids and devices, staying positive.

We each make decisions about how much risk we are prepared to take in our lives, the extent to which we step out of our comfort zones. I like the perspective of author and professor William G.T. Shedd, who coined this quote in 1928: 'A ship in the harbour is safe — but that is not what ships are built for.'

Urban gritty

I seized the moment and went for an afternoon walk beside the busy thoroughfare of Tudor Street in my suburb of Hamilton, in Newcastle. It seemed sacrilege to sit at my computer when the warmth and light wrought a rare transformation of the winter's day outside. As I pushed my red Nitro walker over the neglected pavement, the whoosh of passing cars lulled me.

High above, perched on the curve of its downward trajectory westward, the sun was a white starburst. Even so, its heat was kind to my raised face. A lone crane, stilled mid-work in the distance, reared over a partly built apartment building, and on the roofline of a corner shop, 20 pigeons stood in a haphazard row, silhouetted against the stonewashed blue sky.

Around my home in Hamilton, it's gritty urban. Exercising with the aid of my walker, I call up memories or silently recite poems that I've learned by heart, evoking feelings of relaxation.

This was my street. Wear and tear spoke of its hard life, but I belonged here. Jim's milk bar just around the corner was a magnet for kids and their parents; it sold milkshakes, ice cream of all hues and flavours, and a defiant array of lollies. People leaving the tiny shop exuded an air of satisfaction, barely able to wait to sample their purchases. A man in flannelette shirt, shorts and thongs pulled his toddler's pusher backwards up the median strip, deciding like many before him that he needn't walk as far as the traffic lights to cross the street. Another man, young too, asked me if I was okay as he passed. 'Yes I'm fine thanks, just slow,' I replied.

I sometimes think I'd like to live beside a lake or a grand river, hear more birds, go out each afternoon to watch what was happening on the water, see the changing moods and colours of the weather. With the affection of safe distance, I remember Ballina, the last place we'd lived on the far north coast of NSW, especially the river walks Ken and I took almost daily. Now, from the gym I attend not far from home, I can look out over the Hunter River foreshore and the port of Newcastle. The gliding ships and tugboats lend serenity to the scene, and the still water soothes.

Occasionally Ken and I enjoy the high walkways overlooking Bar or Merewether beaches in Newcastle. When I tire, he'll head off on a longer walk while I find a spot to sit and watch the waves, and the beachgoers. At first my exposure to the sky and water is expansive and enlivening, but before long the restless heaving of the sea disturbs me. If I'm at Merewether, my eyes turn to the quiet ocean pool below me. It's then I know that I'm a lake or a river person.

In his poem 'The Lake Isle of Innisfree', Irish poet W.B. Yeats dreamed of escaping to Lake Innisfree, where he'd build a small cabin to 'live alone in the bee-loud glade'. He wrote of hearing, night and day, 'lake water lapping with low sounds by the shore; / While I stand on the roadway, or on the pavements grey, / I hear it in the deep heart's core'.

I did not get to hear Yeats's lake water lapping the shore but I did connect with some of the highlights from the MetOpera's *At Home Gala Concert*. Old friends revealed themselves from my long-forgotten musical past: *Va, Pensiero*; *Intermezzo* from *Cavalleria Rusticana*. I've saved the site so it's easy to revisit. Listening did bring me joy — my friend was right. I promised myself I'd find the time for more. Music, *and* joy.

Care and focus

Multi-tasking is the signature characteristic of busy parents. My first husband, Dick Cotton, and I both worked full-time, so there was shopping, cooking, cleaning, laundry, gardening, transporting the kids to sport, music and appointments, and a social life of sorts. Most of the time, we managed to keep on the treadmill that was our lives. Occasionally one or other of us lost their footing and toppled off.

Fortunately I have few of these obligations now because I have lost my once-prized ability to multi-task. I take much longer to do things, easily losing my focus. Here's an example. The first thing I do after arriving in our garage after a local shopping trip on my mobility scooter is take out the key and place it in the basket. Next, I unload the shopping from the carry-bag and transport it to the kitchen on that other essential mobility aid, my walker. I make a mental note to go back and press the button to close the garage door and give the scooter a quick clean with an anti-bacterial wipe. Then back to the kitchen to unpack any cold items needing the refrigerator or freezer.

If anyone distracts me from my path, it is easy for one of these tasks to drop out. My mobile might ring, or Ken might ask about a parcel that's just arrived. Or I make a dash to the bathroom. If distracted, I forget to plug the scooter into the battery charger — or if I remember, I must then set the alarm on my mobile, so the battery is not forgotten and over-charges.

All this takes extra energy, the energy of focus and concentration. A narrow vision, shutting out pleasure in the moment.

Then there is my slowness. That's due to neurological damage in my right leg, foot drop and impaired balance. It's not just me moving about the rooms; it's me and my aid. I'm totally dependent on the walker both inside and outdoors. Because of my foot brace, taking off my shoes and socks or changing my clothes are substantial operations.

I avoid buying clothes involving me trying on new garments in a cramped changing room.

The fine motor coordination I depend on for tasks as simple as peeling a clove of garlic, filling an ice tray or locating a light switch often holds me hostage. To take out the washing, I load up a special round basket that fits exactly on my walker and manoeuvre out the sliding doors and across the mini-ramps Ken has installed. The pegs demand my close attention, because if not handled carefully they will slip through my fingers. Bending to pick one up calls for care and focus.

Care and focus. That phrase describes the principles that must govern every move I make. No carelessness, no short cuts, no multi-tasking. No falls. And hold fast to what it is I am planning to do, for fear it will slide away and escape my mind's reach.

Melanoma on the move

Throughout March 2020 Australia's response to COVID-19 was escalating as new cases of infection were reported daily across Australia. Cruise ships such as the *Diamond Princess* in Japan and the *Ruby Princess* in Sydney were disparaged as 'floating Petri dishes of infection'. Travellers flying into Australia had to face the grim prospect of two weeks hotel quarantine. Panic headlines jostled each other in the media.

My husband, Ken, had his own crisis to manage. In the first week of March 2020, a melanoma metastasis was discovered in his brain, through routine MRI surveillance. This was a substantial acceleration. After a flurry of medical appointments, he commenced the first of four immunotherapy infusions of 'miracle breakthrough drugs', ipilimumab and nivolumab. These two drugs work together to help the immune system launch an attack against the cancer.

We pored over the list of possible adverse events that might occur as side effects. The list was long, and it was frightening.

One Sunday afternoon at the end of March, I was reading on my bed, basking in the autumn sunlight streaming through the windows. Suddenly Ken was there, calling for my help, his right arm flailing uncontrollably. He collapsed on the bed, his breathing hoarse. Something was awfully wrong. This must be one of the adverse events we'd been warned about.

Calling 000 for the first time in my life, in my 75th year, was something I'll never forget.

The woman on the other end of the line was measured and calm. I wasn't — how could I stay and keep a close watch on Ken, while getting downstairs to open the front door for the first responders?

In the end, when I sighted the ambulance arrive in the street below, she agreed to my leaving him. I wedged the phone in his hand so she could keep talking to him. I took our small domestic elevator downstairs and pressed the remote control to open the garage door. Then back upstairs again. Ken was still conscious, even holding the mobile to his ear.

Within minutes, a team of paramedics had run upstairs and entered the bedroom — two impossibly tall, lean young men and a shorter young woman with blonde hair tied in a ponytail. They worked on Ken with a calm focus, questioning and soothing him simultaneously, connecting him to oxygen and multiple other pieces of equipment. I was in awe.

Apart from also answering questions, my job was to pack his hospital bag. It was something we'd talked about since he started immunotherapy, but hadn't got around to doing.

I grabbed a large carry-bag and, trembling, stuffed it with things he'd need. The team leader called me back from the bedroom to discuss getting Ken downstairs. They quickly ascertained the elevator was too small to fit Ken and all his equipment. 'We'll call for reinforcements to help us get him downstairs,' I was told.

A few minutes later a smaller vehicle arrived from the ambulance station that was conveniently just a couple of blocks away. Another two tall, lean young men came up the stairs. The teamwork of this newly formed group was organic as they murmured directions and made subtle adjustments among themselves. Ken was manoeuvred downstairs on a stretcher and out into the street where the ambulance waited for him.

I followed in the elevator, out through the garage to the Sunday-afternoon quiet of the street. The reinforcement vehicle had gone; the ambulance team members were talking among themselves, making notes and phone calls. Soon they too were on their way to John Hunter Hospital.

Once Ken was admitted to hospital, the scans and other investigations showed a bleed had occurred from a brain lesion, causing recurrent focal seizures. It was not an adverse event from the immunotherapy drugs after all. Like a stroke patient, one side had been affected — his right arm had lost strength; his walking, balance and fine motor coordination were impaired. As well, there were visual and sensory issues. He couldn't draw a cube or the face of a clock with accuracy. Handwriting legibly was very difficult for him.

Various medications were administered and Ken gradually stabilised. I was unable to visit him because I was recovering from emergency eye surgery for a torn macular in my right eye.

The operation had been performed the day after Ken was admitted to hospital, just beating the state government's deadline for cancellation of all elective surgery due to COVID-19. However, we spoke often on the phone. Ken's older son, Peter, a respiratory nurse in a Brisbane hospital, was in frequent contact with both of us. I felt reassured by his experience and knowledge as well as by his understanding of his dad and how the medications might be affecting him.

Around mid-week, I began receiving phone calls from staff about Ken's discharge. Still vision-impaired and unstable, I was worried I wouldn't be able to care for him at home, especially if he needed help with showering and shaving. Ken insisted he was getting better by the day and would be able to manage his self-care. I thought his medication was pepping him up and giving him an unrealistic view of his capabilities. I wondered about rehabilitation to strengthen his right-side function before he came home.

As the weekend loomed, there was pressure to free up hospital beds and a plan was worked out among staff to transfer Ken to a rehabilitation hospital. He was under the care of a specialist in neurology with a clinical interest in movement disorders and stroke. A nurse phoned to get my agreement. However, Ken was not particularly happy about this decision: he wanted to come home then and there.

Suddenly everything changed. It so happened that my MS neurologist, Dr S, swept in and took over Ken's case.

Ken had met Dr S at various times when he'd accompanied me to the MS Clinic at John Hunter Hospital. She remembered him too. 'Oh, you're the husband, aren't you?' she said when he mentioned his connection to me. 'Now, I don't know much about stroke or seizures, but I know a lot about the brain,' Dr S declared. 'There's not much point having a perfect functioning right side if you're going to be dead in two weeks! Something's got to done about this.'

That was the kind of talk Ken liked. Saying it how it was; action would surely follow. It did. Dr S ordered an MRI that Thursday; later, a Registrar visited Ken and tentatively suggested brain surgery might be the way to go. The rehabilitation plan was dropped.

On the Saturday morning and still at John Hunter Hospital, Ken received a bedside visit from a trio of specialists: a neurosurgeon, an oncologist and a radiation oncologist. There was a new plan. The specialists explained what was proposed and discussed the risks: surgery first to remove the haemorrhagic lesion, then home. Once recovered, Ken would begin stereotactic radiotherapy as a day-only patient to deal with any remnant of the lesion. Immunotherapy would no longer be a suitable treatment because of the acute liver inflammation he'd experienced as an adverse event after just one infusion. Rehabilitation could be an option much further down the track, if necessary.

Everything was happening at speed. Ken was transferred to Lake Macquarie Private Hospital, then to Lingard Private Hospital, where surgery would take place on the Monday. It would be a busy weekend for him: three hospitals in two days.

It all went as planned. When Ken finally completed radiotherapy a couple of months later, there was no evidence of melanoma in his brain or body. That was the best news we could have hoped for, even though we were under no illusions about the likely return of the disease in the future.

I think back to the part happenstance played during Ken's care. He may not have died in two weeks as Dr S predicted had he gone to rehabilitation, but everything we have read since his surgery indicates he would not have survived long. Melanoma in the brain can be aggressive and deadly. It was Dr S's fresh view of Ken's condition that opened a different course of action. She saved his life.

Open eyes

The space I enter is tremulous in the midnight silence. As I move from my bedroom to the bathroom, the way is lit by slivers of light glinting off the stainless-steel bannisters. Automatically, I glance towards Ken's room at the other end to see if his light is on, but all is in darkness. His absence saturates the empty spaces.

Sleep is something neither of us do well. Tonight, the pain in my right foot is excruciating. Usually, I am ready for sleep by 10 pm; I put in my earbuds and choose a 15-minute podcast. Among my favourites are audiobooks from BBC

Radio 4. I was still wide awake when Episode 3 of *A Month in Siena* by Hisham Matar ended. I tossed and turned, trying to ease out the neurological discomforts that emerged to take possession of my body as soon as I lay still.

I'd already taken my medication for muscular spasms, but the usual half a tablet was not enough for the involuntary contraction seizing my foot, curling it inward. The next option was Nurofen, a popular anti-inflammatory my GP had warned me against because of my brush with associated stomach problems. But occasionally, I breached his ban because they really helped my foot pain — and worked in about 20 minutes.

I made myself a cup of weak milky tea in the upstairs landing gallery, hoping it would be enough to protect my stomach. Back in bed, I opened *Griffith Review 69: The European Exchange*, the latest edition. It had arrived in my letterbox that day. Reading print on paper used to prepare me, without fail, for sleep. Half an hour later, the pain was unchanged, and I was not drowsy in the slightest.

Since Ken was in hospital again for a few days, I'd had a light meal that night. Perhaps I was still hungry. I remembered some raisin bread in the freezer; already my mouth was watering. I unplugged my mobile phone, put it in my dressing-gown pocket, and took the elevator downstairs. Ready access to my mobile, especially when Ken was away and I was in the shower or elevator, was critical. If I had an accident or a medical event and was unable to phone for help, it could be many hours — days, even — before a family member worked out that something was wrong.

In the kitchen I made camomile tea and raisin toast and stood, eating, at the counter. It felt good to be upright but it didn't do the trick. I've lost track of the next iterations, but they all failed. I remember that at about 1 am, I resorted to half a sleeping tablet. Because of MS, I am especially sensitive to any medication that goes directly to my central nervous system. It was Saturday next day; I had no commitments, and it wouldn't matter if I was a bit fuzzy. But I awoke at 6.30 am, refreshed.

Going through my morning routine, I reflected on the night. Yes, I had been experiencing pain. Yes, my day had been full-on, starting with a taxi ride to the gym at 7.30 am, two loads of washing, a trip to the shops on my mobility scooter for essentials, and phone calls.

But there was something else, I decided. Each time Ken is away for a night or more, I understand it as the forerunner of what lies ahead. Our marriage is nearing two decades, exceeding the duration of my first. We came together on the cusp of my retirement; he'd already made that choice. Our lifestyle meant we were together 24/7; that's all we knew.

We've talked quite often about the future and his prognosis. Once melanoma gets to the brain it can advance pace rapidly. Until recently, his had been slow-moving. Despite the surgery and wonder drugs that have given him remission, we know that the melanoma will win. Two or three years ago, his life expectancy would have been around six months. Now he's been given a gift of more time, and while it's longer than six months, no one can be sure how much longer.

Last night, when I ventured from my room and found his in darkness, I knew his was a temporary absence. But that knowing could not disguise what my soul felt with a visceral anguish, that one night I would walk out to this small landing gallery and realise that Ken would not be there, ever, again. My soul needed to be awake last night, needed to allow that knowing to possess it.

Needed to allow itself to feel scared about what lay ahead, needed to call on all its strength, and needed to keep vigil for a while longer.

Everyday Zen

The skies have been leaking waters for days; my house cannot withstand the rain's resolve to find a vulnerability, the tiniest fracture, in its structure. For now, a small bucket captures the drips, but Ken doubts a plumber could ever find the breach. On Sunday evening, flash floods hit the suburb where my daughter, Vinodini (Vino), lives — it made the evening news — but she reached home after her weekend shift without mishap. This morning I think about teachers and kids navigating their way to schools all over Newcastle in this weeping deluge and I feel anxious about my grandsons.

It was almost lunchtime when I sat down to write a blog post. Ken had been discharged from hospital the day before and we'd not yet established a routine for his day. Already I'd been up and down in the elevator more than half-a-dozen times. He told me how in hospital he'd ask for something and the harried nurse responded that she'd be back in 10 minutes. With luck he'd see her again in an hour, or more. I understood that nurse.

In the evening I managed to put out our two bins, juggling one in one hand and my walker in the other. Ken said he could have done this — as he usually does — but that was bravado. My next-door neighbours were always saying, 'Anytime, anything. We can help you, in any way at all.' Yet somehow it seemed quicker to do it myself as soon as the rain eased. Ah, there's a fracture, a stubborn independence I've always possessed.

The bin exercise was a balancing one. Weight on either side kept me mainly in equilibrium, feeling only a little precarious. I resisted brushing errant raindrops from my eyes for fear of destabilising myself.

I thought of recent counsel from my friend, and Sydney writer, Cecile Yazbek. 'In Zen we speak of remaining upright on the cushion, all the while being buffeted by storms and demons,' she emailed. 'But for this to happen, remaining upright, we need a strong container, a process, a practice. Zen is but one in this context, your writing is another.'

Carrying out that routine chore I stood upright, I felt strong, and around me was the protective container of a process. My children's father, Dick, used to say that if he kept upright and focused mindfully on the job at hand — doing the dishes, hanging out the laundry — he'd keep at bay the demons of depression. 'One foot in front of the other,' he'd say. A process, a practice, the Zen container of the everyday task.

Throughout my life I've done my share of putting out the bins, but it has become more complicated since I've lost my mobility. Over recent decades with Ken, I've fallen out of practice. There's that word again, practice, a practice. Looking to the future, it may be something I'll be wanting to get better at, work out a cleverer way of managing the cumbersome things. Then again, I might take my neighbours at their word.

CHAPTER TWO

Flux

Pure and simple

'It was the best decision I've ever made,' Ken says, 'moving here to Newcastle. And choosing this location.' My husband has taken to saying this often, especially after returning from another visit to the dentist just two minutes walk from home.

Ken was referring to our 2012 move to this coastal regional city from Ballina, but there had been other moves before this last one.

I'd relocated from Sydney to be with him on his Northern Rivers hobby farm after we'd married late in 2003. It was the second marriage for both of us. I left friendships forged over decades, three adult children and my North Sydney apartment. I took my work with me.

Although I had grown up on a country property, life on the Kyogle farm soon lost its novelty. I felt isolated, cut adrift from many of the most important people in my life. Within a year, the farm had been sold.

Our next home was in Alstonville, a hinterland village sprinkled with lush, cool-climate gardens. However, the allergies that had plagued Ken most of his life worsened here, due in part to a remnant subtropical rainforest adjoining our block. When we found ourselves spending more and more time in Ballina, we decided the coast would suit us better. Once again, we moved, Ken gladly taking on the role of project-managing the building of a new house. We were to spend five years there.

Then in March 2012 Ken and I spent a month in a favourite destination, Spain. My mother, Thelma Tufrey, had passed away the previous winter at the age of 97; for the first time in years, I could travel without the constant tugs of anxiety about what might happen to her while I was away. Still, I knew from experience how destabilising travel could be and I was prone to making out-of-the-blue life decisions after coming home from an overseas trip.

One autumn morning, a couple of months after getting back, I was in the kitchen making breakfast when Ken came downstairs.

'Guess what?' was his greeting.

I looked up from slicing a banana. 'What?' A guessing game was not what I was expecting.

'You have another chance,' Ken said, his voice level. 'Your house is back on the market!'

'My house?' I queried. 'What do you mean?'

'In C------ Street,' Ken replied. 'The one you and Vino inspected two years ago. And the price is a bit lower, but not low enough.'

I couldn't believe it. I'd left Spain determined not to expect or do anything rash. I hadn't imagined it would be Ken who would be thrown off-kilter. I knew better than to interrogate him about how and why he'd changed his mind or why he'd been trawling through the Newcastle real estate pages at 4.30 in the morning.

It was not that house we bought in the end, but the one next door. Both were two-storey, and I knew in my heart that a single-level house would be a far more sensible choice given what most likely lay ahead for me. But Ken was so enthusiastic I dared not risk derailing the decision.

Although I'd lost my mother the previous year, I'd gained two more grandsons, born within a week of one another. There were two in Newcastle — Zeus and Cass — and Samuel in Sydney's northern suburbs. If I wanted to be part of their lives, I needed to be geographically closer. I was 67, with a chronic, disabling health condition and I reckoned that I had until I was about 75 before my capacities became severely curtailed. As well, Ken's melanoma diagnosis was a large unknown in our lives.

Research on successful retirement tells us that moving away from our social networks and everything familiar is not a good idea. I'd tried to retire up north but clung to my health services consulting work as the one thing from my past life that helped me feel connected to the world. My attempts to retire, as well as the move north, were not a success. It is not easy to make new friends when you aren't part of a workplace, or have children at school, or play a sport like tennis, golf or bowls. Thankfully, though, I had found the Bangalow Writers Group, which became my lifeline.

On this move to Newcastle, I thought I would have 10 years at most to make and feel myself at home. Everything fell into place. By 2012, I was fully retired and, serendipitously, my interest in local history had surfaced. I was able to research, write and publish stories, as well as meet interesting people. My mobility held good for the first three or four years; that was enough.

I often say that Hamilton, the suburb where we live, is like a country town within a city. The main street is over a kilometre long and has a wide range of friendly shops and services — most of my life-needs can be met via mobility scooter. This is even more important since Ken's driving has become limited. And given his more complex health issues, it is the excellent range of specialist health services in Newcastle that we appreciate.

In another good decision, but one that also took some time coming, my son Dan relocated from Sydney to Newcastle. In 2015, he purchased a villa just steps from public transport and a small shopping village. Situated equidistant from Vino and us, he values the close connections to his immediate and extended family.

My son David and daughter-in-law Becky in Sydney have completed their family with a sparkly daughter, Grace. They are wise and supportive to Ken and me as we find our way through this new life stage.

Our grandsons in Newcastle have grown up barely able to remember a time when Ken and I were not always nearby. I learned to navigate being close to Vino's family without encroaching on her independence and privacy. She is caring, practical and ever watchful of us both. We've had the privilege of being involved with her boys and their extended family as they grow, learn and face their challenges. They help us remember what mischief, spontaneity and zest for life feel like.

At the age of 75, I feel I am going well and still have things to offer others. The milestone decade of active life in Newcastle that I'd anticipated is within reach too.

Life doesn't always run smoothly, nor is everything perfect. I don't want to make things seem too glossy, because they aren't. But it is good to reflect on life-changing decisions and how they've turned out.

Ken doesn't care to elaborate on why — after two years of indecision — he suddenly decided we should move to Newcastle.

'I knew that's what you wanted,' he says when I press him.

'But I didn't push you,' I insist.

'You didn't have to; I knew. And if I wasn't going to be around, you needed to be with your family. Pure and simple as that.'

The power of one, or two

In these pandemic times, Ken and I are classified as 'vulnerable'. Not only because of age, but also because of compromised immune systems. It's mid-2020 and there are no vaccines yet. During the first round of restrictions in April/May this year, we were cooperative participants, changing habits and lifestyle as asked. In this fifth pandemic month, with Victoria facing Level 4 restrictions and NSW valiantly holding spot-fires of infection at bay, risk is ever-present.

Once or twice a week I go to my local shops for fresh fruit and vegetables, meat, a few groceries, and pharmaceuticals. It cheers me to see familiar faces and chat at a distance. On the way I pass my hairdresser and we wave through the window — I've explained to her that my daughter has taken over her role for Ken and me for the time being.

Among my friends, even those younger than me, there's a similar caution around the hair salon.

Visits from my daughter and grandsons do put us at risk, but Ken and I have agreed that seeing them is a risk we are prepared to take. We moved here to Newcastle to support them; now they help us stay connected to a wider world that, for a time, is mostly off limits.

My small, safely managed gym for people over 65, located in the centre of Newcastle, has at last reopened. That's another calculated risk and after just two weeks I feel the benefit of the targeted exercise. Although the exercise physiologists have kept their jobs through the restrictions, the mood of both staff and participants is subdued.

While Ken is out of action as my driver, I am getting to know Newcastle taxi drivers on the short trips to the gym. Every cab is impeccably sanitised, and every driver has a story.

Luigi migrated to Australia from southern Italy with his family, as a teenager. He is my age but looks a decade younger. He tells me that as an 11-year-old in Italy, he experienced the Asian flu pandemic in 1956–57. There were funerals in their town every week.

'We were terribly poor,' he says. 'It was hard for my parents to provide enough food for us all.'

He remembers a doctor coming to the house. 'He told my mother something I will never forget. He said: *Don't worry about the food. Your children will not die of starvation. But **do not** let them outside the house. The Asian flu will kill them.*'

The story is sobering, and we are quiet the rest of the trip. The doctor's words of advice were incontrovertible and probably saved the lives of Luigi and his family. Unlike COVID-19, the H2N2 strain of Avian Influenza was more dangerous for children than adults. A vaccine was found quite quickly, and the pandemic slowed. But it left its mark on the world and has never completely disappeared.

For me it is not so black and white: there are shades of grey. Since I lost my mobility a few years back, going for coffee with friends at a local cafe has become the staple of my social life. Over the past few months though, my activities outside the house have shrunken drastically. I've met two friends for takeaway coffee in Gregson Park, and one other inside a cafe. I miss the freedom of those much-anticipated get-togethers, the hour of face-to-face sharing of our lives since we last met.

Medical appointments warrant the risk, but sadly, coffee with friends is on the edge. Newcastle has had no new COVID-19 cases for a couple of months, but a recent outbreak at Port Stephens has made people here uncharacteristically fearful. 'Too close for comfort,' more than one person said to me.

I can cope with the hair salon being off limits but every time I forgo a coffee date, I feel a twinge of reluctance. Yet I'm a rational person who knows it takes only one exposure to infected aerosol particles to contract the virus. There have been enough examples in the media of incidental exposure, of someone being in the wrong place at the wrong time.

Ken says I wouldn't survive COVID-19; neither would he. There are only two people who take full responsibility for us as individuals — him, and me.

I wondered why I was having a hard time owning this coffee-date decision, inconsequential as it is in the scheme of things. I decided to stop writing this micro-essay and see if any insights arrived overnight.

Pottering in the kitchen next morning, I was still wondering. Then I asked myself — when was the last time I made a big decision and felt utterly convinced it was the right thing to do? The answer was immediate. I'd made the decision to stop driving.

For some time, my weakened right leg had been becoming harder to move from the accelerator to the brake. I'd begun lifting it over with my right hand — until once I fumbled and only just got it onto the brake in time. I drove home slowly, trembling. With the clarity of shock, I realised that I could be one of those older drivers whose car ran out of control, foot on the accelerator rather than the brake, killing someone's child — or grandchild. It was too terrible to contemplate.

I never drove again.

Another thought that was anathema was being the person to bring COVID-19 into our home. I'd accepted not being able to drive; so too would I adapt to this 'new normal', knowing that a different lifestyle was necessary for us both to stay healthy and safe. I'd found strategies to deal with not driving and I'd find creative ways of staying connected to the people who were important to me.

Throughout the day, I followed the breaking news. Our premier at the time, Gladys Berejiklian, was recommending everyone in NSW wear a mask in situations where social distancing was not possible. She carried one in her pocket 'just in case'. Newcastle's proud record of no new infections over the past couple of months had been trashed. A young Sydney construction worker, probably with some connection here, visited a club and two pubs in Newcastle. He was COVID-19 positive, and hundreds became infected. One person was all it took.

'If you have to spend more than a moment thinking about whether you should do something,' said Premier Daniel Andrews, pleading with Victorians to obey the rules, 'then the answer is no.' The answer is no.

A different perspective

I feel different when I come upstairs to my bedroom at dusk each evening to close the blinds and switch on the lights. From the main window

I look across the townscape, the illuminated bell tower of the century-old Uniting Church centre stage. I always pause there, meditative.

One evening, doing something from the far side of the bedroom, I caught a different perspective. A massive pine stood in silhouette against the fading rose of the western sky. I looked more closely — a Norfolk Island pine, I thought. In the backyard of a house less than a block away, it was more than three times as high as the house. How was it I'd never seen it before in our precinct where mature trees were scarce?

It was as if a gift had been left on my doorstep, unsolicited and undiscovered until I opened the doors of my perception.

I was lucky that day, as I found another unexpected gift upstairs. On the spare bed kept for visiting grandchildren, three soft toys snuggled into the pillows — Puppy, Peppa Pig and Baby Hippo. They were the only three to escape being secreted back to Vino's house by her younger son, Cass, to join his huge clan there. I took a childlike pleasure in arranging the toys on the bed, on the pretext of tidying.

The day of the Norfolk Island pine spotting, I suddenly recognised something had changed.

The toys had moved; they were cuddled up much more intimately. Puppy had a protective arm over the little ones; Pepper Pig had her nose buried in his furry chest. Yes, something *was* different!

I suspected Cass had dashed upstairs on a recent visit but couldn't quite work out when it happened. A couple of days later, I remembered. When Vino was cutting Ken's hair in the upstairs bathroom, I had sent Cass to them with the Dyson mini vacuum to clean up. He must have whipped into the bedroom to check what he thought of as his property and made this quick rearrangement.

The little trio of soft toys spoke to me of a longing for hugs and comfort. In this era of social distancing, grandparents and grandchildren especially have been deprived of this pleasure. I confess, I have hugged my grandsons when probably I shouldn't have. Cass has always been tactile, even as he grows into a lanky nine-year-old, mad about soccer and Fortnite. If he needs a hug, perhaps because something in his day has overwhelmed him and he feels too pressured to cope, I'll give him one. It will be something for both of us.

Let's talk about ... home help

Watching the current affairs program *Insiders* on ABC television was a weekend ritual. One Sunday, after it finished, I was at the kitchen sink washing our coffee cups. Ken had slumped in an easy chair, felled by post-radiation treatment fatigue. He consumed sleep like a starving man; there was never enough to sate the ravening fatigue that refused to leave him. I longed for him to wake one morning and say, 'It's gone! I feel as fresh as air.'

'I want you to know,' I told him, 'I won't be able to keep going like this indefinitely. We're going to have to talk about home help.'

Struggling to sit up straight, Ken replied. 'I don't like that conversation.'

Believe it or not, that response was positive from my perspective. In the past, my husband would have reiterated all the reasons we were fine as we were. Chief among his solutions was me lowering my standards — washing sheets and towels less often, cleaning less, in general not being such a perfectionist. Today, though, he had communicated his feelings while leaving a crack open for the possibility of negotiation.

It had been almost almost five months since our mother–daughter cleaning team stopped coming. That coincided with the first round of pandemic restrictions, Ken's commencement of immunotherapy, and our cleaner's husband receiving a diagnosis of advanced cancer. Because of our vulnerability, it seemed prudent to limit people coming to our house. Surely we could manage for a couple of months?

As the epidemic turned into a pandemic and Ken's capacity to help with household chores lessened, I took on a greater load. Looking back over those months, I felt as if was doing more physical day-to-day work aged 75 than I'd done since I had three young children and worked full-time. My walker had become something of a wheelbarrow, whether I was trundling ironed clothes to the bedrooms, foodstuffs from the garage store cupboard or relocating a pot plant to a sunnier spot in the courtyard.

Ken has always done his share, and more, in running the household. We used to do the supermarket shopping together but in recent years he took it over himself. When the lifting became too much for him, we changed to online delivery. He continues to maintain the computers and all things mechanical and electronic, as well as ensuring a stream of the latest movies and television series for us to watch after dinner. Since his most recent surgery, he has difficulty reaching down, so he can only unload the top shelf of the dishwasher. Even that helps. He'll begin a task like hanging out some washing but then fatigue may overtake him, and he'll struggle to finish the task.

It's difficult to find information about how long this fatigue will last. It could be anything from months to years, continuing long after cancer treatment has ceased. I remember well from my early MS flares being suddenly overwhelmed by a suffocating weight and barely able to lift my head.

Both Ken and I have been assessed by officers from My Aged Care so we can receive services under the Commonwealth Home Support Program. Ken was particularly impressed by Paul, who, as a former nurse, showed a deep appreciation of the challenges ahead. My assessor, Kathryn, was equally insightful.

Kathryn updated herself on my situation when Ken's melanoma metastasised to his lungs and brain. Because of COVID-19, she and I spoke on the phone. 'Ken has been your carer,' Kathryn said, 'the one able to do the harder physical tasks day to day and help you. Now the roles are reversed.'

It hadn't quite happened yet, but it could soon. She'd seen it all before.

'There is help available for you,' Kathryn assured me. 'Just phone.'

Soon after, while Ken was in hospital recovering from brain surgery, I did just that. I'd gone into a panic about cooking. Worried about my clumsiness and deteriorating knife skills, I decided to register for delivered meals. I knew two women who used that aged care service and were happy with it. They still bought fruit, salad vegetables and staples, but the service provided their main meal of the day. Delivery was in frozen packs, once a week or fortnight.

I pored over the menu listing and marvelled how far things had come in a culinary sense since my mother had Meals on Wheels in Bingara, a small country town in the north-west of NSW. I planned to order meals for four weeks so Ken and

I could test out the service. He was sceptical. I fantasised about how much time and effort I'd save by not getting in so many groceries or preparing and cooking meals. Someone told me it would change my life!

Sadly, not true. The meals were small and unappetising. While I don't consider myself an adventurous cook, my meals are tasty, healthy and generous. I cancelled the authorisation for the service, citing my reason as a reaction to the additives in the meals — true but not the only reason.

Once back to my chopping and cooking routine and being super-careful, I thought about all those older people who had no option but to depend on these meals. How could one survive on such small portions without becoming malnourished?

I'd learned my lesson but was glad I'd tried. I'd keep going for as long as possible, simplifying our daily lives and even trying to be less of a perfectionist. But one day, Ken and I *will* have that home help conversation.

Return of the midnight cat

As I turn each illustrated page, I am surprised how few words are under each softly cross-hatched picture. It's been nearly four decades since I'd read this book to my youngest child, but after all this time, the story can still bring me close to tears.

An archetypal story of change, *John Brown, Rose and the Midnight Cat* by Jenny Wagner tells of the relationship between Rose, whose husband died 'a long time ago', and her dog, John Brown. Through the simplest of word-and-pen pictures, we discover their shared life and love for one another. 'We are all right, John Brown,' said Rose. 'Just the two of us, you and me.'

Into this comfortable, routine life comes the midnight cat. He is the disruptor. First, he lurks in the garden, unseen but sensed by Rose, ignored by John Brown. She wants to give the cat some milk; John Brown can't accept this. When Rose is safely in bed, he goes out and draws a line around the house. He tells the midnight cat to stay away. 'We don't need you,' he says.

A power struggle between Rose and John Brown ensues. Rose secretly leaves milk for the midnight cat; John Brown secretly tips it out. Dog and cat argue, each in their own corner. Then one morning, Rose does not appear in the kitchen to get John Brown's breakfast as usual. When John Brown goes to see what's wrong, Rose tells him she's sick. 'I'm staying in bed,' she declares. 'All day and forever.'

John Brown has plenty of time to do a great deal of thinking. Finally, it dawns on him: he knows what will make Rose better. What's more, it's within his power to give it to her — if he can bear to let go, make a little room.

As the midnight cat is allowed into their home, things change — but not that much. Rose gets up and sits by the fire as before, the cat making himself comfortable at a cat-like distance on the arm of the chair opposite. Now they are three, but John Brown still has pride of place beside Rose. The midnight cat purrs.

My first black eye

It happened mid-morning. A delivery of groceries ordered online had arrived. I'd just returned from upstairs where I'd taken the last few items to be stowed in our bathroom. The elevator had stopped a fraction above its usual level; I stepped out, caught unawares by the longer step down. Everything seemed to happen in slow motion, as I crashed first into the walker, then the office chair, until I lay flat on the floor, face down. Blood spurted, spattering my favourite blue shirt.

I was able to pull myself to my feet, staunch the blood flow with tissues and get to the bathroom to clean up. The furniture had buffered my fall and the only damage seemed to be a small cut below my eye. I didn't call Ken until the scene of the disaster had been put to rights and my cut covered by a Band-Aid.

I couldn't conceal the real damage from him for long. Soon my eye swelled up and injured blood vessels flamed red. My face was shocking to behold, even as bruising set in.

The performance of the elevator was reviewed but no fault was found at the time. (Months later, the offending fault was located during a routine service by the elevator technician.) For the present, however, responsibility came back to me: I must be even more careful and focused.

The Mayo Clinic via Google provided directions for treating a bruised eye, which I followed scrupulously. On the fourth day, I covered the affected part of my face with foundation and concealer and ventured out to the pharmacy in Beaumont Street, the main street of Hamilton. The next day, when I met my friend Vicki Coughlan, who'd cycled over from a nearby suburb, the concealer wasn't needed.

A week after my accident I had an appointment with my optometrist, Lloyd Turner, to check if everything was alright with my eyes. Like most in my care team, Lloyd is in mid-career. We shared an interest in Hamilton's local history. I showed him the photo Ken had taken of my battered face.

'Were you wearing glasses when it happened?' he asked.

'No,' I replied, 'I don't wear them in the house except for watching television.'

'Then you were lucky. They can add to the injuries and, of course, smash so there's the cost of replacement.'

'I think I've had a lucky escape in every way,' I told him after he had given me the all-clear and the consultation was over. 'But then, what's that really mean? It's no guarantee that the first time will be the only time. That there won't be a next time when I might not be lucky.'

Lloyd, who had risen to retrieve my walker from the corner, nodded in understanding, a troubled expression shadowing his face.

'It's what's ahead, what's next,' he said slowly. 'None of us knows.' Gently, he passed the walker to me so I could rise safely from the chair.

Feel and hear

People who know me well remark on my calmness. I'm an introvert, drawing my energy from quiet activities, introspection and interacting with one or two people at a time. I've learned the skills of an extrovert that had been so necessary for the work I used to do. I've also been called a harmoniser — a middle child who seeks the middle way, the reconciler and peacemaker. These attributes, too, were essential for my work. But this doesn't mean I'm not vulnerable to the churn and distress of an altercation.

I work hard to minimise conflict in my relationships, and that may not always be healthy. Sometimes it feels good to burst out with what I really think, insist the other wait and hear me out. The danger is when my explosion misses the target; perhaps I've been seething inwardly over something, someone else crosses my path and gets in the way of my disproportionate outrage. That must be the fate of many a call service customer representative when the caller finally gets through.

One day Ken and I had what I'd call 'a spirited dispute'. Afterwards, I went to my room to rest, but found it hard to calm down. Then I remembered something I'd read in the book I'd just finished, *Room for a Stranger*, by Australian writer and general practitioner Melanie Cheng.

Andy, an international student from Hong Kong, is living rent-free under the Homeshare Program with Meg, who is 75 and alone. His responsibility is to provide 10 hours of assistance to her each week. Andy suffers from anxiety and is becoming overwhelmed by the challenges of his studies and life in general.

At one point in the story, on the brink of a panic attack, Andy recalls a process the university counsellor had taught him.

> Three things he could feel. Three things he could hear. He could feel the pillow beneath his head, the wooden bedframe in his hand, his hair resting on his forehead. He could hear a motorbike storming past the house, the distant cry of a child, birds chirping

> outside the window. He concentrated
> on his breathing.

Gradually he calms and begins to think of practical action he needs to take.

I close my eyes. Three things I can feel. I feel the weight of a pain across my forehead. I feel my stomach roil. I feel the back of my head against the pillow's softness. Three things I can hear. A buzzing in my head. The muffled horn of a cargo ship entering the distant port. A pigeon cooing in the courtyard below. I concentrate on my breathing.

The simple mindfulness process works for me too. It completely diverts me from going over my grievances in my head. They were trivial anyway. I rest for a while, then rise and venture out into the sunny afternoon for a walk. The animal rescue shop where I buy free range eggs is about to close early but the kindly volunteer hands me a dozen as she locks up. 'The back-rent from the lockdown is killing us,' she confides. 'But we're determined to keep going. We must. The animals need us.'

CHAPTER THREE

Shedding Skins

When lost is found

'Since I lost my mobility . . . ' It's a phrase I often use, but I wonder if it's true. I do still have my mobility: I can walk (with an aid); I have good upper body strength; I am reasonably flexible. What, then, have I lost?

A few years after my diagnosis of MS, I noticed I couldn't traverse the distances I was used to without sitting down for a rest, or maybe two. This was especially so in the buzzing Chatswood malls, where sometimes I would go at weekends with a very long shopping list for the family. Now I know that was MS fatigue and, over time, I learned to pace myself so I could achieve my modest goals.

When Ken and I lived in Ballina and I was semi-retired, we walked most afternoons along the foreshore of North Creek, an arm of the magnificent Richmond River. We aimed for The Point, where these waters met and the incoming ocean waves were tamed by the breakwater, perfect for learning to surf. There we rested on the rocks and watched for dolphins.

Then I started to say, 'Let's just go as far as the bridge today,' and the Missingham Bridge became our goal. In time, I'd elect to sit on a bench some distance before the bridge and tell Ken, 'You go on to The Point; I'll wait and rest here.' My capacity shrank.

For a while after we moved to Newcastle in 2012, I was able to walk to the Hamilton railway station — a kilometre each way — with a rest. It wasn't long before I ceased that route in favour of shorter ones around streets closer to home, but I was still taking walks for exercise. Two years later, towards the end of 2014, I was using a cane for support.

Then followed a marked and progressive decline over 2015 and 2016. I knew that most of my MS lesions were on my spinal cord, demyelinating the nerves that carried messages to the rest of my body. I was a likely candidate for mobility and balance issues later in life. An important milestone was reached when a private physiotherapist noted what she thought were early signs of foot drop in my right ankle. The diagnosis was confirmed by a physiotherapist at John Hunter Hospital, and I acquired my first ankle–foot orthosis. The aim of this type of orthotic is to hold the foot rigid so the toes don't flop on the ground and cause a fall. The incipient weakness in my right side became far more obvious and soon I was walking with a limp to compensate. My balance worsened.

I progressed to more sophisticated orthotics and even trialled a state-of-the-art Functional Electrical Stimulation device. A cuff, worn around the leg just below the knee, contains electrodes that deliver an electrical shock to the nerve that goes to the muscle responsible for lifting the front of the foot. If all one did was stride along a straight path all day, wearing the cuff would be fine, but electric shocks are fired off at the slightest movement. Working at the kitchen counter or ironing, for example, involved countless small movements back and forth, side to side. I found the barrage of shocks unbearable.

I began using a walker to give me stability and minimise the risk of a fall. Now I wonder whether I have accepted my decline at the hands of this chronic disease too readily. Was there something else I could have done? I've been to rehabilitation services, physiotherapists, exercise physiologists, orthotists . . . complex disorders like mine in older people don't hold much attraction for medical practitioners because there is no quick fix. Or any fix, really. As disability increases, we are largely left to our own resources with occasional interventions when some specific health issue crops up.

It may be time to reframe how I think of myself. I've not lost my mobility; *I have a disability that affects my walking*. That sounds better. My greatest loss, however, is my ability to drive: my agency. Travelling beyond my suburb to meet a friend for lunch, attending a writers festival, a poetry reading or a meeting, shopping at leisure in a department store — such outings now are complicated, and rare.

It's ironic that as I mourn these losses, the pandemic is snatching away the opportunity of such gatherings from so many of us. Not just the pleasure of participants but, more seriously, the very livelihoods of business owners. While we have been lucky here in Newcastle, no one is untouched.

As I reflect on the past five years, years that have seen the full manifestation of the disability that has been lying dormant in my body for decades, I realise I do have agency after all — it's the power to claim and shape the narrative of my life. And in so doing, to find its meaning.

I wonder how I have journeyed to the place I now find myself. Have I made things unnecessarily difficult, the way I've searched for solutions, perhaps denying the inevitable? Have I come the long way round, taken the road less travelled, eventually to reach acceptance? Maybe so, but the journey has been an important part of the process. It's the way I do things.

Life in short bursts

Springing out of bed in the morning, fully upright, loose-limbed, not a creaky joint to be heard — it's a distant memory. Instead I ease myself from under the bedclothes into a sitting position and wait for a minute or two till I feel my blood circulating. Perhaps I massage a spasm out of my calf muscles. Then, onto my feet . . . and I'll spare you the remainder of my morning reality tale. Still, I'm fortunate because after a while I am walking.

When I was first diagnosed with MS in 1997, people with whom I shared this news reacted in quite different ways. It is hard to know what to say, whether to sympathise, to be a Pollyanna, or something in between. My accountant hastened to tell me of a friend of his with MS who said the best thing about it was getting a disability parking sticker.

But it was the response of my friend, researcher and career coach Dr Susie Linder-Pelz that really helped me. Susie knew someone — the late behavioural scientist Dr Erica Bates — who'd been her senior at the University of NSW. 'I always knew Erica had MS,' Susie told me. 'It didn't seem to affect her ability to work. But I do remember that at every opportunity, she'd rest her legs. "Putting my feet up," she'd say.' Susie described seeing Erica working from home on her bed, happily surrounded by a profusion of research papers, books and notes.

That's the picture I've kept in my mind all these years as I do my share of putting my feet up. Because of that essential rest — especially of vulnerable legs — I was able to continue my consulting work until my late 60s. That's when we moved to Newcastle, and I began a different kind of life.

Stiffness is one of the most common symptoms of MS. It often goes with spasticity. I can sit at a table having coffee with a friend for an hour. After that, unfolding myself to stand must be undertaken slowly and with care. An hour and a half is my maximum: that precludes the cinema or a concert. I can travel by car, plane or train for almost two hours before needing a standing-up break: that longer period is probably because those seats are more comfortable than a cafe chair.

In the 1970s, I took up yoga. I explored the teachings of the Indian philosopher, educator and writer J. Krishnamurti, travelling solo through Asia with a book of Hindu scriptures — the Upanishads — in my bag. Yoga continued to be part of my life, in one form or another, until now.

I used to have a stretching program adapted from yoga to meet my specific needs and stave off stiffness. Once on the floor on my yoga mat, a sense of calm washed over me. It was my time, my space, my respite. It was a conditioned reflex from all those years of practice, still part of my muscle memory, even though there were times I lapsed.

Is there a link between physical and mental flexibility? Does a flexible, supple body mean one is more likely to have a more flexible way of thinking? In the 1990s, I studied metaphysics, and my teacher certainly believed it did: the understanding that the body and mind were intimately connected would eventually become mainstream. Present-day yoga practitioners claim that its practice can enable psychological flexibility: the ability to adapt, shift perspective and choose the best course of action from competing ones.

A variety of research studies are demonstrating how physical activity, especially in older people, can improve cognitive flexibility, originality, even creativity. It has also been associated with better balance and lower risk of falls.

While Ken and I await the arrival of our new cleaner, after six months of managing it ourselves, I am gratified to read that even short bursts of light activity such as housework have been associated with a reduced rate of brain volume shrinkage in older people.

That's a lot of incentive and encouragement for me to keep up my gym visits, as well as daily sessions at home on my NuStep cross trainer. It is placed boldly in my living space — I pass it multiple times each day, never ignore it and will never regret purchasing it.

So, short bursts are my thing — and I'll still *rest my legs* because rest is what fuels my next little activity, housework included. And it's staying on my feet, being active, doing things, however modest, that keeps me in the game.

Making space

One late afternoon in 1993 when I was living with my three children in Willoughby on Sydney's lower north shore, an electrical storm struck. Next morning, quite by chance, I noticed that the largest and most beautiful tree in my garden had acquired a small split in its trunk at the V-shaped junction of two branches.

Over the years, I had resisted all attempts to curtail the eucalypt because it created a leafy haven around the back deck. Now there was obviously something very wrong. I found a tree surgeon in the *Yellow Pages*, phoned and he agreed to come the next day.

Early next morning, daughter Vino woke me with the news that one of the branches had fallen. We rushed out. By some miracle, it had fallen exactly into the gap between the deck and the studio where her brother David lay asleep, oblivious to the threat from above. The flower garden I'd been nurturing was saved because the thick branch just happened to be shaped to arch perfectly over it. Another garden bed was not so fortunate, but the damage was limited.

Then I looked skyward at the branch that formed the second half of the V. Precariously, it reared back over my house and that of my neighbour. Its other half was no longer there to balance it. I dared not imagine what the neighbours would think when they saw it.

With growing anxiety, I phoned the tree surgeon to ask him to come sooner. No answer. I tried to work in my home office with that fallen branch lying prostrate against the French doors, its leaves brushing the glass. Every time I looked up, I heard the words in my head: *Trust. Trust. Trust.*

The tree surgeon didn't even turn up at the time he'd originally promised, later in the day. After multiple phone calls, I found someone who would come at 6.30 next morning. The kids and I went to bed hoping against hope that there would not be the slightest breath of wind that might sever the branch and send it crashing through the roofs of two houses.

There wasn't. The removal of the tree went smoothly next morning. I repaired my gardens, bought new seedlings from the nursery and planted them out.

Within days, it was as if the whole garden had a new life. The lawn, always straggly beneath the huge eucalypt, grew thick and lush. Tiny flowers I'd not known existed popped out and bloomed. We revelled in the morning sun that had never reached the deck before. 'No,' I told the relieved neighbour. 'We don't think we'll plant a replacement. We never would have removed that gum if this hadn't happened. But now it has, we can see the benefits and we like it this way.'

Simpler still

'**You can get** rid of that — and that — and that,' I instructed Ian, who'd come on his annual visit to tidy up our three courtyards and front garden. I had pointed to one pot with a tree that had died; another overgrown with weeds having long lost its original tenant; a pile of empty plastic pots stacked near the air conditioner. 'I need to simplify these courtyards,' I declared. 'If it's not doing well, it has to go.'

'You sound like my wife,' Ian replied, grinning. 'From the start of the pandemic, she's had me clearing stuff out. In fact, I think I'll call you Tracy!'

'I should meet her' I said, laughing. 'I think we'd get on!'

Some hours later the courtyards had been transformed and Ian's truck was fully loaded. The lemon trees had been carefully thinned, no longer reaching over the front wall to drop fruit on the footpath. One of them, its growth stunted by the other trees, had been removed. On the south side, a variegated creeper that had flourished far beyond its guiding lattice and well into our neighbour's territory was now pruned into submission. Spiky no-name plants heading for the skies had been brought under control and looked agreeably stark against the grey courtyard wall. The passionfruit vine had been trimmed lightly. A clutch of wooden stakes was stowed out of sight because, Ian said, 'You never know when they might come in handy.'

Outside the gate against the front wall is a thriving rosemary bush, grown far too big for the narrow garden there, and encroaching on the footpath. As a herb it complements roast lamb, but we only eat red meat occasionally these days. 'Maybe dig it out, do you think?' I asked Ian. 'Oh no! I have clients who would die for a bush like that!' He paused. 'I'll just tidy it up for you. Don't worry, it will be fine,' he added soothingly. I imagined him thinking, *Phew! I just saved that one!*

This house had appealed to Ken because it hasn't a blade of grass to mow. There is still plenty of scope to grow things in the courtyards, and over the years, potted plants have multiplied. Yet every plant needs water, fertiliser and care; courtyards need sweeping and cleaning. For me it's all about maintenance.

Like our mother, my three sisters have green fingers, creating beautiful gardens wherever they've lived. Regrettably, that's not me. But I do love bursts of summer annuals, the fragrance of herbs and lemon blossoms, and the leafy companionship of trees. It's just that these days it's logistically and physically harder to keep up the cycle of planting, watering, removal and renewal.

It occurs to me that if we choose to engage with anything that has life — a plant, a person, a pet — something within us is called forth. Responsibility. We discover what it is to honour another. And even a back aching from weeding the garden, a nest of cat fur on the sofa, or that phone call from your friend who unerringly rings just as you are sitting down for dinner affirms your connections in this world. These things become offerings, a kind of grace, a cause for gratitude.

Fishpen Road

On the sixth morning, I woke as if from a long, arduous journey. My head, at last, was clear from the onslaught of the flu. Thoughts arose, floating towards me fully formed, no longer shredded by my fever.

Ken had become ill first. There was no mistaking what was ahead, leaving Canberra on the second leg of our road trip to Merimbula. Once he started sneezing, he didn't stop. Somehow, he stayed at the wheel, resolute in his misery. It was inevitable that, being confined with him in the car for three hours, I'd catch the bug too.

We were not to know this would be our last trip away before COVID-19 landed in Australia, grounding its citizens. In our holiday villa, Ken helped me unpack the grocery staples we'd brought, then stumbled to his bed. We'd stayed in this two-bedroom 1980s villa by the lake the year before, so it was both familiar and comfortable.

The downside about our location was distance from the shops. I had relinquished my drivers licence as worsening MS immobilised my right leg. Now Ken was out of action, I was stranded. The lively main street was a 15-minute walk over the bridge — nothing to most people. For me it was impossible without the mobility scooter that ensured my independence at home.

When Ken rallied temporarily, he was able to make short forays out by car for pharmaceuticals, fruit or a takeaway meal, occasionally bringing back a coffee and muffin each. I became ill a couple of days after our arrival, and although I had a fever, my attack was less severe.

Our plans for morning excursions to the towns and villages we'd enjoyed so much on our previous visit — Eden, Pambula, Candelo — were binned. We wouldn't get to visit the once-pristine coastal community of Tathra, still recovering after a fiery conflagration had consumed more than 100 buildings the previous summer. And in Merimbula there'd be no browsing the richly stocked newsagent for books or board games for the grandchildren; no flicking the clothes racks to find that elusive top for an upcoming celebration;

no lazy coffee mornings at a favourite cafe overlooking the water.

As we battled our infections, being kind to each other, preparing simple meals and drinking copious water, the days passed.

It was early April, the sunshine at its softest, the air playful with watery breezes. Sleek magpies strutted the lawns surrounding our villa; wattlebirds cackled and squabbled as they searched the trees for nectar.

From my chair on the porch, I became familiar with the ebb and flow of the tide, always surprised when the spare frames of the oyster farms rose like ragged monsters from the deep. Our street was Fishpen Road; in the 1930s fishermen used to net salmon here, penning them inside the lake against the causeway. Very likely the Yuin people used the natural features of the lake for a like purpose, long before the salmon fishermen.

At low tide herons, curlews, terns and sandpipers fossicked for living food along the mudflats. Pelicans rested comfortably on whatever vantage point took their fancy. And several times a day, small planes buzzed over the town, carrying passengers between here and Sydney or Melbourne.

Each morning and evening, I ventured out along the lakeside paths, steadied by my Nitro walker. Schools had resumed; the late stragglers were friendly. We chatted idly as travellers do. I returned to share snippets of news with Ken, lying in his darkened room groggy with flu medication.

After breakfast, my eyes protected from the dazzling lake, I sat outside reading *Griffith Review 63: Writing the Country*. The fine spare font on the parchment-coloured pages echoed the bleached cattle bones of my country childhood. Through every essay, it seemed, I could hear the groaning of our land, ravaged by climate change. On my lap, I held the book with reverence, even tenderness. I felt like a tuberculosis patient recuperating in the gardens of a Swiss sanatorium, prescribed rest, fresh air and sunshine. An invalid, like my country, only it may never recover.

On the seventh day of our holiday, my head clear, I walked much further, this time away from the lake. I pushed the walker up a long slope to a cafe opposite the beach. I felt as if I'd escaped, proud of how far I was managing to walk. Even a bit excited. The cafe was on a corner and already crowded as I steered around the tables towards the counter. A young woman with a toddler anticipated my need and adjusted the stroller to make room for me to pass; a couple in perfect leisurewear pulled in their chairs. I ordered a coffee and found a table where I could park without blocking the passageway. Even that momentary hassle, common to those of us with walking aids negotiating busy places, didn't dampen my joy at feeling normal. The downhill walk home would be easy.

I found Ken at the table, showered and shaven, eating a tomato sandwich. He was keen to know what I'd seen. 'When it cools down this afternoon,' he told me, 'we'll go for a drive.'

In the grip of social media

I've been clinging to my Facebook accounts when I'd really love to close them both. These days I rarely post, but I like to check my feed for community activities and news. I use old-fashioned email and phone to keep in touch with friends and family, and occasionally FaceTime, Skype or Zoom. Never have we had so many options for communication other than face-to-face. Does this mean we are happier and more connected?

I did have a reason for hanging on — a personal page is necessary for me to have a community Facebook page to promote my *Hidden Hamilton* blog. I began that social history blog in 2013, soon after moving to Newcastle. I have a personal Ruth Cotton Facebook page, and a Hidden Hamilton Facebook page.

I closed my blog in January 2018, although it is still online. It is preserved for future readers by the State Library of NSW in PANDORA, part of the Australian Web Archive. Since my *Hidden Hamilton* activity has come to an end, I no longer need a Facebook page. Sounds logical, doesn't it? So why all the agonising?

I think I might be worried that if I close my Facebook accounts, I'll lose my friends and followers. I have email addresses for everyone who is important to me, but what about thousands of other followers? Won't I be letting them down?

Being realistic, I am sure they will have well and truly moved on and found other more active social media to follow. I will write one final post to say what I'm doing, thank them, and remind them my blog is still available.

And I'll close my LinkedIn account. After all, I retired from real work several years ago, so it is just vanity that keeps me there.

Do I still need my personal Facebook page? Like most people, my friends include people I know in real life as well as others I've met in cyberspace. The original reason for my connection with many of the latter has escaped my memory.

Occasionally I've seen people post a notice to say that they are refreshing their list of friends and if anyone would like to remain a friend, to please send a Personal Message. I imagine that's an effective filtering process. To be blunt, a cull.

Some decisions are emerging. I'll close my Hidden Hamilton Facebook and LinkedIn accounts. I'll put my personal Facebook page 'on notice'. South African writer Antjie Krog quotes her mother, the Afrikaans writer Dot Serfontein, in *A Change of Tongue*, reflecting on how in the past it was reading fiction that gave us access to a different, larger world, but no more:

> But nowadays this larger world is
> incessantly present in your yard and on

> your stoep (verandah) and in your guest
> room and in your kitchen, it takes up so
> many seats at the table, it always has a
> whole mouthful to say about your food.
> Because of television and newspapers,
> you are now saddled with this other
> world. And you want to get rid of this
> other world, you wonder desperately how
> you are going to overcome it. Intimacy
> with your own world is the one thing that
> enables you to survive this ever-present
> other world.

It is this intimacy with my own world that I now seek to explore more closely.

I've experienced how liberating clearing out 'stuff' can be. Even more importantly, I've discovered how stepping back from some of the commitments that encroach on my life creates space. I've learned that allowing freed-up time to rest like a fallow field for a month, or six, or even a year allows something else to present itself and win the right to my time and attention. That 'something else' is usually something I could not have imagined when I'd opened the space.

I have a growing desire to peel away the inessentials from my life. I don't want to leave documents, possessions and trails in cyberspace for my husband or kids to puzzle over and dispose of when I've gone. Everything I keep must have a purpose. As I clear the ground of my life, what will enter?

I didn't have long to wait for an answer. I scribbled a few notes about this reflection and wrote a post for Hidden Hamilton's Facebook page, explaining it would be taken down at the end of July 2020. The post triggered a wave of generous comments in appreciation of my Hamilton work. So far, so good.

Then, in the serendipitous way things happen when they emerge from deep consciousness, the idea of a new blog came to me. It surprised me because I thought I'd done with blogging.

My Hamilton blog and books had been other people's stories; this blog would be mine. I would call it *Morning Pages: My life with multiple sclerosis and other uncertainties.* Through it, I would communicate in a deeper and more authentic way with the people who are important to me.

I'd honoured the past not just by writing about Hamilton as it once was but also about my own family's history. Now it was time to write about my life, in the present.

Girona dream

Every bit as infectious as the Delta variant of COVID-19, it swept across NSW. Restrictions on the way we lived our daily lives were being lifted rapidly; the scent of freedom made us giddy with anticipation. Yes, it was the travel bug.

I noticed it first among my classmates at the gym. One couple rebooked for Christmas 2021 at Norfolk Island, after getting as far as Sydney airport on their last, failed attempt. Another keen traveller had already disappeared up the north coast with her daughter. The 20-something exercise physiologists joined the 70-year-olds in excited exchanges of dates, itineraries and accommodation tips. Then it spread to my suburb, as a friend with family in Melbourne seized on the promise it would open for the Melbourne Cup and made her booking.

Even Ken and I caught the bug. We'd last travelled overseas together, to Italy, in late 2015 and I had accepted that there would be no more adventures. I was using a cane then, and Ken arranged wheelchair assistance for me at every airport.

Now, with daily announcements about Europe reopening to tourists, attractive international fares and easier quarantine arrangements, Ken did what he does best. He searched for an accessible apartment in Girona, a Spanish medieval city we'd not yet visited. The apartment had to be 'in the buzz' yet quiet, with an elevator, plenty of light and memorable views — preferably a church tower and some greenery. We'd avoid trains, hiring a car and driver to take us from Barcelona to Girona, and stay there a couple of weeks. When Ken found the perfect apartment, even a bakery and cafe downstairs, it seemed possible. We'd make one last, grand effort.

Over the next couple of weeks though, doubts began to set in. Articles appeared in the online media about international travel being far more stressful than before the pandemic, with the cost and inconvenience of pre- and post-flight COVID-19 testing being a major deterrent. As Ken and I visualised the complicated logistics of every section of our trip, we realised that neither of us was as able or competent as we'd been even in 2015.

Back then, Ken had been able to manage baggage for both of us and cope with the unexpected events that inevitably happen when one is on the road. Now he tired easily and handled stress less well. Although I am physically quite strong, my impaired balance places me at risk, especially in unfamiliar circumstances. If one of us became ill or hurt, the other may not be able to rescue them. We needed someone to travel with us, sound of body and mind.

'Let's face it,' Ken observed, 'we're damaged goods. Both of us.'

I had to laugh.

Reluctantly, we shelved our Girona dream. No harm done, no bookings made, just some indulgent fantasising. I suspect we were not the only ones who went to the brink during those early, heady weeks. And it was fun while it lasted.

CHAPTER FOUR

Tracks in the Sand

Skies clearing

On the last day of winter, the threshold of spring 2020, the sun was bright but not yet hot as three of us sat at a table in Hamilton's Victorian-style Gregson Park. Tea was poured from thermoses, and fruit cake from the local grocer shared. Talk was cheerful, the minutiae of daily life: fruit bats eating my fallen lemons; Bev's last harvest of snow peas for the season; Jan's new supplier of delivered meals. When I said my goodbyes, I felt flushed with the heat that had ambushed me as the morning passed.

As the weather warmed, passionfruit began to ripen and fall from the very top of our vine, now almost on the roof. Each day, I collected a single fruit, as delighted as a child finding an egg in a chicken coop. Then they fell in twos and threes, until one morning, I found five in a scattering over the paving. I gathered them with care, adding them to the others to fill the bowl to its brim. There they rested untouched for a week, gleaming in rich purples and greens.

The tumbling of the passionfruit, their sudden release from the tight grasp of the vine, felt like a sign. I'd been shedding old skins, making space in my life; now what had been blocked or thwarted was free to move forward.

I've worn hearing aids for maybe 20 years, updating them every five or so. My last pair, bought in 2015, were the most expensive and the least satisfactory. Then Ken's reduced capacity for driving forced me to rethink every relationship with a service provider that required car travel, and I began looking for a new audiologist closer to my home.

When I met Glynis McPherson, I warmed to her immediately and knew she was my future. My new aids — a different brand with the latest technology — elegantly integrate into every function. Whether in person, over the phone, via radio or television, my hearing is transformed. Conversations in noisy cafes are so much easier. I've realised how in the past, small anxieties moved in on me, squeezing my breath as I entered a situation where hearing might be difficult. Glynis and Oticon have changed my life.

Hearing impairment is in my family. My father lost his hearing, just like his father, his brother and five sisters. My mother retained hers until defeated by very old age, but her father became deaf relatively young, as did my mother's sister. Among my cousins, there's a scattering of hearing impairment.

I was grateful, too, when, later that same day Ken arrived home from his three-monthly visit to his oncologist. The appointment was to review the reports of an MRI of his brain and a whole-body PET scan. They would show if his melanoma had recurred anywhere.

'The news is . . .' began Ken, putting his cap and bag on a chair, 'nothing to see here. Nothing happening, no treatment recommended. Watch and wait.'

'Oh, that sounds good,' I responded. 'And what about that small lesion in the brain?'

I meant a new, unidentified lesion that had been found in his June 2020 scan.

'Not active,' replied Ken. 'The single infusion of immunotherapy I had must have zapped it. Still there, and most likely a metastasis, but it's doing nothing.'

Ken had been quite concerned about that lesion, so this news was very good. His extreme fatigue had begun to lift; he was exercising daily and feeling better. Now, until his next round of surveillance in three months, he could consolidate these gains, allowing his body to recover further from the onslaught that is cancer treatment. Two personal wins for us then. Small, but no less remarkable than the glow on those passionfruit.

Beyond ourselves

Research backs up the idea that being part of something larger than us gives meaning to our lives, makes us healthier and happier. 'Something larger' can be having a job that we believe makes a difference, being a parent or grandparent, or religious faith. But I have a nagging sense that something is slipping away from me.

My life has been rich with meaning over many decades. I've worked in fields such as HIV/AIDS, rehabilitation and Indigenous health; my consulting work over 20 years brought me into contact with health organisations and services at points of deep crisis. I've been able to 'make a difference'.

I've maintained an enduring connection with the children's home in Kandy, Sri Lanka, from whence my first husband, Dick, and I adopted Vino, a little sister to our two sons, in 1983. In my retirement, I've volunteered in primary schools and aged care facilities; I've coordinated a parents' mental health support group and a writing group, and I've immersed myself in uncovering and writing about the history and heritage of my suburb, Hamilton.

Through all these years of raising my family, coping with vicissitudes such as MS and family illnesses, I've found spiritual sustenance through nature, wide reading, friendships and shared rituals.

So what's bothering me?

As my life has become more constrained, exacerbated by the pandemic, I have felt the domains of meaning in which I'd once moved so fluidly being lost to me. It's much harder being physically present with people and causes I care about. More of my energy is diverted into taking care of myself, Ken and our home.

Yet in the early summer months of 2020, I feel normality being restored, ever so subtly. My grandsons are visiting safely; Ken and I are, once more, helping with their school projects.

Cass's speech development plateaued several months ago, and a new approach was investigated and put into place. 'Team Cassius', comprising parents, grandparents and therapists, is working hard to give him the best possible start in life. When I was deciding on a career, *speech therapist* was on my list. I know now that I would have lacked the persistence and patience needed to help a child achieve such long-term goals — but by helping Cass I am getting a chance to try it out anyway.

School holidays have come and gone, and the end of an incredibly disrupted school year is just around the corner. The days when I sat with children who had never experienced a parent hearing them read have long been replaced by encouraging my own grandchildren to read and choosing new books with them. I no longer visit lonely nursing home residents but help in supporting my brother in a far distant facility. From time to time, I find him books and DVDs and we communicate via my sister-in-law's text messages. Seated at his bedside on her loyal and regular visits, she shares the details of his quiet days, and relays snippets of local news that have caught her fancy.

I upbraid myself that I am not doing enough, that my engagement with the world is shrinking. But I know that the time for the grand gesture is over. As I follow global news and politics, I grow anxious about what the future holds for the generations following us, especially for the children.

The media bombards us with stories of suffering, of persecution and exploitation. Like others, I need to be careful that my interest remains healthy and not disabling.

Now I shield myself as best I can; I gather my loved ones close, reinforcing my sense of safety, belonging and feeling beloved. I focus on the small generosities that are within my gift, counting them and marvelling at their number. And at their heart, I find the meaning that is my sustenance.

Come the day

Suddenly the jacaranda trees across the street were in bloom. On the edge of effusiveness, the lavender flowers danced out of two showery days just passed. The grand old trees had survived many a Council pruning; they were far too large for our cramped street. But when they performed each November, casting an extravagance of confetti over the footpath and into the street, the neighbours' complaints were silenced.

And there was another joyful happening at the weekend. Grandson Cass was staying overnight while his mum celebrated her 40th birthday. A winner of the US presidential election had not yet been declared; like so many others, Ken and I were on tenterhooks. As the three of us sat around the dinner table the topic came up. Gulping mouthfuls of lasagne, Cass took over the conversation.

'Joe Biden is going to win,' he declared. 'He's got 270 votes, but Trump only has 214.'

I stared at Cass in surprise. 'Joe Biden' had rolled off his tongue with the familiarity of an old friend.

'Trump won't admit defeat, though,' he went on. 'He's going to go to the Supreme Court!'

'How do you know all this?' I ventured.

'Oh, I watch the 7 o'clock news,' the nine-year-old replied. 'Most nights.'

'And who have you been talking with about this?' I pressed.

'No one,' he said, grinning. 'Just myself.'

With any other nine-year-old, this conversation would not necessarily have been unusual. But since being diagnosed with a severe speech disorder at the age of three, Cass has worked hard every single day to forge links between his brain and the muscles of his tongue and jaw to articulate hundreds of individual words. Through those years, his capacity to generate and practise the patterns of speech has lagged. Conversation between us has been largely question and answer, although of late we have been starting to have more complex exchanges.

The surprise of that dinner table conversation was not just Cass's knowledge but also his clear articulation and self-confidence. A primary goal of his therapy is to be able to speak so he can be understood by his teachers, family and friends. That doesn't seem a great deal to ask, but for him it is huge.

Through my journey with Cass, I discovered so much about this amazing capacity that seems to occur naturally — speech. For each of my three children, it happened on cue. When Vino, his mum, came from Sri Lanka as a three-year-old to join our family, she learned English. It seemed to happen with ease. Until something goes wrong, we barely give the acquisition of language a second thought.

As the jacaranda tree is primed to bloom in spring, so, too, is each child genetically programmed to stand on two feet, to walk, to speak. That seems like a miracle.

It's an even greater miracle when Cass's determination — encouraged by those who love him and guided by caring professionals — gradually pays off. When he is finally able to communicate his needs, feelings and opinions and be understood by others *every time* he speaks — that will be the pinnacle of his achievements.

And with all this talk of miracles, there's a small one I'd like to ask for: to live long enough to see that day.

Saving love for what is close

In her poem 'I Save My Love', Nebraska poet Marge Saiser evokes for me the way my life has become gentler, more inward, more enwrapped in the familiar. Not just during the pandemic of this year but as age and disability weave their subtle limitations into the texture of my daily life:

> I save my love for what is close,
> for the dog's eyes, the depths of brown
> when I take a wet cloth to them
> to wash his face. I save my love
> for the smell of coffee at The Mill,
> the roasted near-burn of it, especially
> the remnant that stays later
> in the fibers of my coat.

I, too, save my love for what is close, for what stays, for what lasts. A pink mohair throw rug gifted to me over 30 years ago by my mother-in-law Edna Cotton stays in a cupboard close by, ready for that unexpected night chill. I might have preferred a different colour, but the rug holds in its feather-light fibres such intensity of Edna's affection that tears prick my eyes as I write this.

The upper level of our home is lightly decorated with photographs of children, grandchildren and moments from overseas trips that Ken and I have shared. A few special gifts are in evidence, too — mementos that have survived the rigour of my regular cleansing of possessions. I could update the photos — especially the ones of people — but I want them to stay as they are. A passing glance is enough to trigger the neurological pathways in my brain; the rush of dopamine-induced warmth through my body is its own reward.

I remember Edna's sister, our Aunt Lorna Menzies. A former maths teacher who'd never married, she poured all her love into her grand-nephews and nieces. In her 80s, Lorna had a severe stroke and was placed in an aged care home. I used to visit her, sometimes taking the children, and often found her reading the same book. Her pleasure in it remained undiminished. I know now she was reading a comfort book: a book that was personally significant to her, its words, sentences and pages deeply familiar. They brought her solace, allowing respite from a reality that was, for her, confusing and uncertain.

I, too, am consciously gathering books I've loved — by writers such as Alex Miller, Helen Garner, Elizabeth Strout, Shirley Hazzard, Atul Gawande, Sebastian Faulks, Colm Tóibín, Frank Moorhouse, Orhan Pamuk, Pat Barker, Georgia Blain. Among them are books I'll read again and again. Less and less, I seek the groundbreaking or the innovative, just the familiar trusted voices with no surprises.

It's happening with movies, too. There's a special file on my computer titled *Nursing home movies.* The file name may be tongue in cheek, but it's also a precaution against the possible time when, anchored in one place, my days will be long, and I'll want to watch films that soothe me.

I used to nurture a wide network of relationships and strove hard to maintain regular contact, often travelling far afield to do so. Now I accept that this is unrealistic. At such a complex time in my life, friends and extended family members are self-sorting according to the level of communication they feel comfortable with. I am surprised by some of those choosing to step closer, as I am by some who move gently back.

The important thing is that the burden of obligation I once felt to people in my life has become something much kinder. Love has no bounds, but my capacity does; like Saiser, I save my love for what is close.

Threads of connection

Summer extinguished spring as smartly as a candle flame is snuffed; suddenly 60 bushfires raged across NSW and temperature records tumbled. Sydney Airport registered 43°C on the last day of November 2020. Australia had just experienced its warmest spring and its hottest November on record.

The centre fell out of my week, the penultimate before Christmas. Ken strained a muscle in his back; every appointment we had that required him to drive was rescheduled for the New Year. I missed my Tuesday gym session and my grandson his always-anticipated overnight stay. What would happen in the vacant space that had been created?

Across the street, one of three villas had been silent, blinds drawn, the owner's car and small dog missing for weeks. 'Where's Julie?' I wondered to Ken. I knew she had a respiratory condition so I concluded she must be in hospital.

While Ken was lying flat on his bed with a hot water bottle under his back, Julie's blinds flew up and for a couple of hours, a stranger came and went. 'Someone is cleaning,' I informed Ken. Later that day, I noticed pieces of lounge furniture stacked against the wall under the carport.

Next day, the furniture had gone, and a rubbish skip appeared in the empty carport. Another mystery person, or perhaps the same one as before, filled it then disappeared. The gates were shut against the empty carport, and the kitchen blinds, once again, were tightly closed.

I told the story to Greg, our podiatrist, on his six-weekly visit. He nodded. 'Pretty much every week,' he said, 'I get at least one email saying one of my clients has passed away. Sometimes it's a surprise; sometimes it's not.'

Greg went on to explain that in the large retirement villages he visits, the giveaway sign of a resident's passing is tradespeople entering a house. 'Management refurbishes every home before it is put back on the market. New carpet, curtains, refrigerator, dishwasher, the lot.'

An air of forlorn finality hovers around the villa across the street. We wait, now, for the real estate agent to appear.

In the meantime, marking the mornings of my hollowed-out week, the postie trickles Christmas cards into the letterbox. I rail against this: how many years have I been trying to reduce the number of cards I send? I began my reduction by keeping only people over 80 on my list and emailing everyone else. I have a particular antipathy to what I call 'empty cards', those containing only the most superficial of messages. What a waste! I want to know *how you really are.*

Then there are other friends, seen infrequently, who do the opposite — enclosing a Word document that is crammed with details of the achievements of by-now three generations.

Among my email recipients are those with whom I'm in regular contact anyway. For them I add my good wishes to an end-of-year email in a way that shows how I value their friendship. For those with whom contact is less frequent, it's a chance to briefly catch up on the highs and lows of the year. And some, like a dear friend whose vision no longer gives her the option of reading anything short or long, I telephone.

As my empty week reveals the multiplicity of ways people choose to communicate about Christmas, I recognise that this is, after all, the real point. We each have different preferences about how we'd like to wish others well and I need to have my antennae tuned to that. Whether someone wants to send me a Jacquie Lawson ecard, an exquisitely textured reprint of an artwork, a Merry Christmas Santa card with a two-line message, an email, an SMS or WhatsApp message — I'll accept it with grace and reply in whatever mode I feel like at the time. People who send *actual* cards do it because they like to and want to. It really is the thought that counts and I'll stop being grumpy.

The recent happenings across the street have set me back. They are a reminder of how tenuously we hold the routines of daily life — or perhaps they hold us. It's a fragile hold, ever at risk. A neighbour has just told me Julie has been moved to residential aged care. I didn't know her well but noticed the pride she took in walking her little dog early every single morning, spot on 7 am. No doubt she wrote and posted a bundle of Christmas cards this time each year to special people in her life. I wonder if she'll manage to do that now?

Nurturing these gossamer threads of connection in our insecure world is a privilege, not a chore. Like an incoming tide, that knowing fills my week.

Recipes for calm

I needed a mundane task, something to ground me, calm me. In the lead-up to Christmas, anxieties in our household began to mount. NSW had been doing so well in managing COVID-19, then everything changed. One case led to another and the whole of the Northern Beaches LGA was locked down to contain the outbreak. Greater Sydney was on alert.

Even after a happy and COVID-safe Christmas, my mind still jangled. Looking for solace, I turned to my recipe collection, which I'd planned to digitise as a New Year's project. One quiet afternoon I carried two ringbinders into my office and switched on the scanner.

Over the years, I'd culled recipes that I thought looked interesting but had never tried. Others kept their place, having been tried once not very successfully but retaining potential given a tweak or two. Recipes signified different fads and phases of my life: vegetarianism, low calorie, the Mediterranean way of eating. My folders were the slimmest they'd ever been, but this round, more recipes would go.

After some internet research, I decided to use Microsoft's OneNote. It was plain, functional, and looked simple enough. Recipes could be scanned and uploaded as pdf files, cut and pasted, or their URL added as a reference. I checked with daughter-in-law Becky. 'Yes, sure. That would work well for recipes,' she assured me.

Calories to the wind, I began with *Cakes*. In that section were several I'd typed up from Mum's recipe book after she'd passed away in 2011. Recently Ken had become keen on a recipe called 'Charlie's Favourite Drop-on Cakes', a staple my mother used to make for my father and any hungry men who happened to be helping him on the property. A simple butter cake mixture with added sultanas and citrus peel, these palm-sized cakes melted in the mouth when warm from the oven but didn't stay fresh for long. Then two recipes for date loaf: my mother's, with sparing use of butter, and my sister Jan's, more generous. How cleverly Jan used empty fruit cans in which to cook her mixture, so she had three novelty loaves to freeze for that unexpected visitor. And calorie overload — Amanda Hinds's chocolate brownies! I remembered meeting this local architect for the first time, her passion for heritage, and my unabashed indulgence in her cooking.

Surprisingly, it was not the mindful process of digitising but the sight of recipes in my mother's handwriting that calmed me. Years back, clearing her things from her Bingara unit when she moved to a care facility, I'd found an exercise book full of her recipes. Pages were faded and torn, some falling out, others nibbled by insects. I'd scanned most of her recipes, and though her book did not survive, images of her carefully written recipes had. Now I saved the pdf under the heading *Cookbooks*.

Scrolling through the pages, I see that my mother's clear and well-formed handwriting reflects her logical mind and organised approach to life. It feels reassuring, calm, competent. She was always there, in the kitchen of the country home in which she'd lived for 60 years. She offered food to all-comers to smooth life's rough patches. The cooking process must have been, for her, a meditation. Her recipes were recipes for calm.

I'll never finish my project if I go on like this! So many recipes evoke memories of people I've loved and valued. Like my first husband, Dick, his mother, Edna, and Aunt Lorna who helped me so much as a young mother; treasured activities like Ken and grandson Cass making mini-custard tarts; recipes from new friends like Amanda, Julie and Kathryn, made since moving here. For a couple of hours each day over the next three days, I work my way through the sections — soups, vegetarian, meat, biscuits and more. A few aspirational recipes are permitted to remain — *still looking good, yet to try.* And when I come across a recipe in someone's handwriting, even if I don't particularly want that one, I scan and save it in my digital collection. They've gifted me not just a recipe but something of themselves.

The task takes nowhere as long as I'd thought it would; it isn't even 2021 yet. At the end, my office rubbish bin overflows with discarded pages and the two empty ringbinders are stowed in the cupboard.

Next time I need to refer to a recipe, I'd pull it up on my iPad in the kitchen. I am satisfied with my end-of-year work. Best of all, like a garden refreshed by falling rain, I am calm.

An attitude of kindness

The crowd from the church spilled outside, merging with those who'd not been able to find a seat at my father's funeral. Country funerals can be large but my father's funeral was huge.

The Anglican church in the small north-western NSW town of Bingara is neat and well kept — chocolate-brown brick with white trim. When I enter its austere space, I feel a lump in my throat. This June day in 1990 was no exception. But it is what happened outside the church that I remember clearly.

A young woman approached me, a man by her side. She wore a dark shirt buttoned at the throat, a V-necked jumper and skirt. Her clothes were simple, chosen for the occasion, but I could see immediately she'd be more comfortable in riding gear.

'I want to thank you for everything your father did for us,' she said after introductions. 'He helped us when we were struggling on our farm; he took our horses when we couldn't feed them during the drought and returned them in wonderful condition. He helped us in so many ways.' Her words had poured out in a stream; when she paused for breath, the young man reached for her hand.

'He believed in us,' he said, his blue eyes blurring.

Similar stories were recounted many times that day, as I moved from one cluster to another throughout the gathering. Still in a state of shock myself, I'd barely recovered from the long drive from Sydney. My father, Charlie Tufrey, was almost 80 when he died, the lymphoma he'd had for some years spreading to vital organs. Many in the crowd were of his generation. What struck me though, bringing me firmly back to earth, was the number of younger people there — all ages, but most in their 30s and 40s.

Charlie was the youngest of eight siblings and stayed on the family farm to work by his father's side. That was his destiny, and he did a good job. But his passion was horses, and it was serendipitous that he could collect, breed, train and show horses while working the large sheep property.

Like his pioneer father, James, Charlie was a highly skilled horseman and trainer. Over the decades since his death, I've come to understand that my father had another, different attribute: the capacity to mentor others. He loved people as much as he loved horses, and their potential captured his imagination. I doubt he would have described himself that way, but I recognise it in him because this mentoring gift has been passed on: to me, and to my sisters, who have had long and dedicated careers as teachers.

One of my own mentors once said it didn't matter much what career we chose — we'd find ways of using our gifts. That's been true for me — in the many different settings in which I've worked, I've always found time and opportunity to mentor others.

'Mentor' sounds like a modern word because of its popularity in the human resources field. In fact, it derives from the character Mentor in the Greek epic poem *Odyssey*, attributed to Homer. It has come to mean one who imparts wisdom and shares knowledge with someone less experienced.

Thinking about the origins and present-day usage of this word though, I wonder whether much of what is done in the name of mentoring might be at its heart just one thing — an attitude of kindness.

In these pandemic times, we are being urged to be considerate of the young front-of-house employees checking our vaccination status as NSW opens to a freer way of living. 'Treat them as family,' says newly elected NSW Premier Dominic Perrottet. 'They could be your son or daughter, or your neighbour's.'

Patience, a smile, a considerate act — every life we touch with kindness becomes part of our legacy in the memories of others. As the winter sunlight blessed that country churchyard, and people remembered my father, I discovered this as if for the first time.

Lifting our eyes

'**The overwhelming feeling** was that someone had pushed the pause button; I stopped, seemingly drawn into someone else's story. But the stronger feeling was of waiting, holding my breath, of looking always to the future. It wasn't true. A lot happened.' These are the words of my friend and former colleague Gray Sattler in his New Year's email from Bangkok, looking back on 2020, the year just past.

That's how I felt too: waiting for the next set of COVID-19 numbers; a lockdown announcement; borders closing then reopening; the nail-biting US election results; someone's medical reports. Most of those things were far beyond my control but some affected people I care about. Despite my daily emotional investment in 'someone else's story,' life went on.

The defeat of Donald Trump in late 2020 and the modest ascension of Joe Biden had felt like a global tectonic shift, its sound like a sigh of relief across the earth. Not the man, Biden, frail like the rest of us in his age and humanness, but everything he stands for and has aspired to in his lifetime — decency, compassion, equality, cooperation.

Dan Rather, an American journalist and former news anchor, is 89 years old. His daily writings on social media platforms such as Facebook and Twitter can be depended on to give courage, reassurance and hope in these most difficult of times. With wisdom and gentleness, he enjoins us to lift our eyes from our feet to the horizon.

On New Year's Day in 2021, he wrote about 'the carnage of 2020 that will literally bleed over into 2021' and the 'great undercurrent of uncertainty and hardship encircling the pandemic globally'. With these prescient words, he referenced the political situation in his own country. Then on 6 January 2021 came the unimagined, unprecedented storming of the Capitol building in Washington. An underscoring of the already deep and troubling divisions in US society; a crucial turning point in the history of its democracy.

Dan Rather draws attention to the relative privilege that so many have enjoyed at this time through easier life circumstances. He calls on those of us with this privilege to shoulder a greater burden, to hold on to hope for the sake of others. 'We need to be better, to do better, to act better in 2021,' he pleads.

The social constraints on my daily life about which I complain occasionally are insignificant in comparison with the 'easier life circumstances' I enjoy: groceries delivered to my door; a place to exercise in safety; a companion with whom to share my daily life.

My MS is stable: no surprises. Ken is in remission for now: we are grateful. Friends and family are good communicators, and we stay connected through whatever medium works best — sharing ideas and happenings, recommending books and films. We encourage each other in fresh endeavours and through unexpected troubles. Grandchildren stay healthy, learn, achieve, have fun and bring delight to my life. How privileged I am.

Here in Australia, thousands of healthcare and care workers, testing and laboratory staff, politicians and media people show up to work night and day 'to keep Australians safe'. That's a cliché but it's also a massive reassurance and our great good fortune. Everyone else benefits from their endurance and sacrifice.

On 25 January 2021, it will be one year exactly since the first case of COVID-19 was diagnosed in Australia — in Victoria. Over that time I've been expecting the worst. I anchor myself in Dan Rather's challenge: *to shoulder a greater burden, to hold on to hope, to be better, to do better, to act better in this year ahead.* I think about what I can do, how I can be more creative in the way I respond. I listen to NSW Premier Gladys Berejiklian conclude her morning briefing: 'We want people to feel more optimistic about the future,' she says. Hold on to hope.

There is no doubt that here in Australia the incredible collective effort of the past year has helped to shore up the deep strength and hopefulness of the communities we live in. Every positive thing we as individuals do or say adds to the global store of goodness. It's a way of passing on what Dan Rather has given his readers — inspiration for us all to keep going, to keep giving, to keep looking ahead.

CHAPTER FIVE

Befriending the Brain

When the air hits your brain

'You ain't never the same when the air hits your brain' is the First Rule of Neurosurgery, as described by American neurosurgeon Frank Vertosick Jr. in his medical classic *When the Air Hits Your Brain: Tales of Neurosurgery.* This maxim sums up the subtle changes that can occur after cranial surgery, changes we began to record after Ken's first craniotomy in March 2020.

I've told how, after few days in John Hunter Hospital following a seizure at home in 2020, Ken was operated on to remove a lesion in the left parietal lobe of his brain.

A biopsy confirmed it was melanoma that had metastasised and haemorrhaged. Soon after, he commenced a series of stereotactic radiation therapy treatments as a 'mopping up' exercise in case surgery had missed something.

Treatment to reduce inflammation in his brain (high doses of corticosteroids), the surgery and the radiation all took its toll, along with the single infusion of immunotherapy he'd had before the seizure. Ken was aware of residual damage to his functioning, but it has been very difficult to pin each deficit to a specific cause.

One of the first deficits we noticed back then was at the meal table — managing a knife and fork, especially with his right hand. Ken was finding it difficult to bring his fork or spoon accurately to his mouth, often missing and spilling food on the floor. He could dress himself — mostly — though aiming his hand at the right armhole for his shirt sleeve was a challenge at first. It was not unusual for him to painstakingly button his shirt, only to find he'd matched the buttons wrongly and had to start again. He could tie his shoelaces, although he had to concentrate and was slow. For the first few weeks he depended on me to help him put his socks on.

Keen to get back to helping with chores such as unloading the dishwasher, Ken met hazards. He'd accidentally knock over glasses and drop plates, making him frustrated and cross with himself.

This cluster of deficits, we learned, could be attributed in part to the fact that the lesion had been in the left side of the brain. That meant that the opposite side of his body was affected — his right arm, hand and leg were weak. Most interestingly, the lesion had been in the parietal lobe. Simply put, that's the centre that integrates a whole range of sensory information among various modalities — somatic sensation from the skin (pain, touch, temperature, motion), as well as visual and auditory information that gives us the spatial sense necessary to analyse where in space our limbs are located. The latter is proprioception.

That's why it was hard for Ken to put his shirt on, avoid the wine glass on the kitchen counter, correctly direct his fork to his mouth or insert a key in the keyhole. Proprioception enables us to do such things without a second thought.

We noticed a curious thing when he tried to slide his right hand into his trouser pocket. It's something we do automatically, without looking down to visually locate the opening. But Ken always missed the first time, then had to look down.

Because visual information also gets integrated in this amazing little switchboard in the brain, Ken could relearn certain things by looking, when, in the past, visual cues hadn't been necessary. Take shaving, for instance: he used to always shave while showering. He was able to relearn this quite quickly by shaving in front of a mirror. So, too, correctly locating the turning indicator in the car or unlocking the front door.

When my driving days were coming to an end, my right foot was finding it increasingly difficult to locate or differentiate between the accelerator and the brake. The numbness of my foot and damage to critical nerves prevented sensations reaching my parietal lobe, so I couldn't accurately analyse the position of my leg. That was serious.

Many of us have found our handwriting has deteriorated since computers have taken over our lives. Ken's is no exception, only now it is worse. One of the first things he did once out of treatment was to buy a special trackpad for the computer as he found it difficult to manoeuvre the mouse. That helped for a time, until he recovered.

The difference between Ken and me is that because of the nature of his 'injury', he has been able to improve. Mostly, I haven't. The best I can do is hold my ground against the natural decline of ageing.

He regained functionality in most of these areas over the ensuing 10 months, but I continued to be watchful of him. Faithfully following his exercise program gradually helped to retrain his brain as well as increase fitness. Ken was very happy to resume some of the handyman tasks he used to do, though he paces himself as he suffers fatigue and lacks stamina. He can now draw a perfect clock and cube: the test he was given by a psychologist soon after his seizure showed these objects grossly distorted.

This whole experience has taught us how vulnerable the brain is to even the slightest injury. Dr Vertosick is right — you can't open the brain, remove a bit of this and that, and expect everything to be the same. But then that's the other thing about the brain — an amazing ability to change, adapt, make new connections and heal itself. While things mightn't be the same after surgery, the brain's neuroplasticity will be working away in the background to restore and recover as much functioning as it can. That's a truly remarkable phenomenon to witness.

Memory matters

'**The details escape** me for the moment,' I say, 'but the gist is . . . ' I'd noticed myself making this excuse from before I retired, only now the details are on the run far more often. I've always used to-do lists and a diary to track my commitments. Although paid work no longer floods my days, these strategies are more important to me than ever. A Google calendar has taken over the diary, and Ken regularly asks Amazon's cloud-based voice service Alexa to help him out with the temperature for the day or a reminder for something he wants to do later. Neither of us can write very legibly by hand, though we scrape by with our typing.

As self-appointed 'Entertainment Officer', Ken organises a variety of movies and television series for us to watch in the evenings. Yet he finds it near impossible to keep their names in his head. On the spot, he asks me what we saw the previous night, or what he'd just told me we would be watching this night. I try to be patient, reframing his questions as a useful test for my own memory.

Ken's memory is far better than mine when we try to remember the name of a village we'd visited or stayed in during our overseas travels. He has a brilliant visual memory, so while it might take a few minutes for him to remember the name, he then gets a mental map of exactly where the village is located. And if we happened to stay there, the route into our accommodation!

Skills acquired over a lifetime seem to take longer to attrite with age. Reflecting his past career in electronic engineering, Ken is still good at maintaining our phones and computers as well as solving the problems that inevitably arise in our technological environment. I've noticed, though, that he is slower, wanting to proceed in a careful, sequential way without interruption. He regularly urges me to acquire new computer-based skills, and I gently offer the excuse that I plan and organise most other things in our lives.

I had been worried about my own memory for some time, knowing that it was not as good as it used to be. I was finding it more difficult to speak fluently, hold my own in a fast-moving conversation, grab the right word in an instant.

I'd tried the Lumosity computer games my friend and Hunter poet Kathryn Fry had recommended, ones that challenge memory, reflexes and peripheral vision. I struggled with the games and made poor progress. Over time I decided that instead, I'd do something to stimulate my memory that I really enjoyed, something that would be a wellspring of lasting pleasure.

I was pleased when the idea of memorising poetry came to me. Kathryn helped by sending poems, and I found that the 'scaffolding' some poems possess helps the memorisation process by providing hooks from one word, idea or image to another.

I learned not to be too hard on myself when the perfect word chosen by the poet eluded me. I discovered the inner joy that flowered as I traversed the lines of a poem I loved, usually as I pushed my walker around Hamilton.

It was when I began attending the gym in the Honeysuckle precinct of Newcastle that my mental functioning really sharpened. Through twice-weekly classes, both the exercise itself and tracking what I was doing on the Finnish-designed state-of-the-art SmartCard machines kept me focused, extending body and mind. And at home I practised not rushing to the Google search bar every time my memory failed me: instead, I waited, trusting, giving it a chance. After all, it is ageing, too.

75 and counting

'**You scored only** 29/30?' my GP Dr B exclaimed in mock horror, sliding into the spare chair in the practice nurse's office. He was skimming the Mini-Mental State Assessment I'd completed. Nurse S broke in. 'It was the season question. She thought it was summer, not spring!'

'Think how hot it's been,' I argued in weak self-defence.

'Oh no, it's been freezing — we had to get the doonas out again for the girls last weekend,' responded Dr B. He'd relaxed, seemingly glad to be momentarily free of the straitjacket of back-to-back patient appointments. And to be one up on me.

The cognitive test I'd done was part of an hour-long Medicare Health Assessment for Older Persons 75+. Dr B had raised it with me months before, explaining they were looking to cover all eligible patients in the large practice.

'It includes a cognitive assessment,' he'd told me, just a little gleeful, as he knew how I felt about that. 'But . . . it's just to get a benchmark.'

I agreed to the whole thing, on the day answering endless questions about my life, health and wellbeing. Could I shower myself? Cook? Manage my finances? Did I care for anyone else? Did I receive support services in the home? How did I sleep? Had I had a fall in the past three months? Did I drive? Drink alcohol? Was I incontinent? Then a raft of questions designed to find out if I was depressed.

There was a master list of medications and vaccinations to check, as well as details of a string of medical and allied health professionals I consulted from time to time.

The 75+ assessment overlapped with the Chronic Diseases Management Plan, which is completed for me four times a year. Thankfully, the two reports could be merged. And although we'd treated the cognitive assessment in a light-hearted manner, the issue is serious. Not that long ago, I'd left the iron on. Before that, it was the gas burner on the stove top, so low it was barely perceptible. Ken noticed both and I felt mortified. Is it ageing, or something else? There was no specific question to pick up such lapses.

I know of a few people who'd benefit from the 75+ assessment, especially the cognitive test and depression questionnaire. It is understandable, though, that spouses, partners or friends worried about the state of mind, capacity or incipient dementia of loved ones might be fearful of broaching such sensitive issues, let alone suggesting consulting a GP.

It seems a comprehensive assessment for everyone 75 years and older is a good thing because it's all in for everyone. No one is singled out. The patient must consent so has a choice. It's bulk-billed under Medicare, hence no reason why all eligible patients should not be taking advantage of it.

When the nurse had finished administering the assessment, she'd called in Dr B to sign it off. Before he did, we three spent some time discussing whether there were any gaps in the care I was receiving, any unmet needs or health issues not being addressed. That's the purpose of the assessment, a structured way of identifying needs and issues that might have been missed.

I suppose this mega-assessment will become a regular experience for me every November from now on. Next time, though, I'll remind myself of the season before I go!

Building respite

In search of respite, I sat down to write. During the past week, activities and unplanned commitments piled one atop the other. I'd enjoyed everything and adapted readily to hasty rearrangements. At the end of the week, I was running on empty.

The details don't matter, but here's a sample. Vino's car developed a fault and she borrowed ours; her son Cass's specialist appointment led to a medical procedure from which he needed to recover. A local osteopath had to be found for follow-up. We took care of our grandson; then his older brother visited. One of my comments on our precinct Facebook page drew unexpected interest and the rush of comments and messages needed attention. I took taxis to my gym sessions, making the trips more complicated.

All this has made me think about respite. In 2020, the combination of COVID-19 isolation and Ken's cancer treatment prompted my Aged Care case worker to ask if I'd like respite. 'Someone to take you out for the day,' she suggested. 'Or even just a wander round the shopping mall.' I thanked her, telling her not just now. But I'd not forgotten the offer.

Not long ago, Vino had taken me to check out a new Coles supermarket, part of a recent development in her suburb. She was pleased with its easy accessibility, wide aisles and choice of fresh produce. I enjoyed my morning outing with her, just as I enjoy the company of fellow classmates at the gym. I never dreamed I'd come to depend on such simple pleasures, getting me out of the house.

I found myself looking at my crowded calendar, thinking, 'I just need to get to . . . say, Wednesday night.' But Wednesday night came and the list for Thursday was even longer. And so on. I felt as if I couldn't get my breath.

Perhaps I am seeking a different kind of respite. It doesn't take much for anxiety to take over, anxiety about how I am going to do all that I expect of myself. One thing gets ticked off, then another one rises to the surface. Before long I find that anxiety is a constant bodily reverberation, a state I come to accept as normal. I feel like a hummingbird, beating my wings at an ever-faster pace just to stay aloft. Until it gradually dawns on me that life is losing its lustre.

I've always been someone who gets things done. In retirement, I've continued to have goals and aspirations, though rather different from those that filled my working life.

Anxiety and high achieving go together: some of us are conditioned from childhood to feel intense satisfaction when things get done — ticked off. We tend to do them sooner, not later, to experience that pleasure hit. As more tasks flow into the vacated space, we keep going and before long become successful because we can be depended on. That can be the road to what's known as 'the respectable addiction' — addiction to work. I know about this.

While time out with friends or a shopping expedition can be valuable respite, for me it's rather more nuanced. I like to think of respite as something we've trained ourselves to build into every single day of our lives. The words *train* and *build* have been used deliberately, suggesting that this takes time.

I've come to think of respite as consciously pausing after each anxiety has been settled or each goal achieved. Not looking around restlessly for another objective to dominate my days. Not rushing ahead to snuff out the next lurking anxiety by 'doing'. Pausing, taking the time needed to create a respite experience for myself.

In his book *Status Anxiety*, Swiss-born British philosopher (and high achiever) Alain de Botton warns against exactly this: replacing one anxiety with another, substituting one desire for another. Achieving our goals promises us respite and resolution that they can never deliver. Which is not to say we shouldn't have goals, he says, but our lives will be easier, less anxious and driven, if we build this awareness into our strivings.

It's the nature of these small but emotionally rich periods of respite that matters. Often they're empty space. Now, there's a challenge — to allow that space to stand alone and untouched, at least for a while.

A reading life

My library book, its newly laminated cover gleaming, slid into the returns chute. Published this very year, praised by leading reviewers, the debut novel failed to capture me. A worryingly common occurrence these days.

All my life, I've found stimulus and solace in equal measure in books. Even in my busiest years, holding down a job and with three young children, I'd find time to read. Reaching for half an hour away from the clamour, reading was my respite.

Now something's changed. I continue to borrow books from the library, buy them on Kindle or occasionally from Hamilton's go-to independent bookshop. I read reviews avidly and choose accordingly. Often, though, the review draws me in more than the book itself and I end up disappointed.

Reading novels has always taken me to places never dreamed of, opened my mind to ways of living, thinking and being that I could never have imagined. Showed me ways of using words I can only aspire to. Reading I know is a discipline, a muscle to be trained and conditioned. Time must be set aside for practice, like learning a musical instrument.

But now I find dense lines of print hard to focus on, and a 400-page book heavy in my hands. Why is it that often I can't connect with what I'm reading? Is it the writers of our times, an age difference, or am I losing my empathy, my capacity to put myself in another's shoes, my willingness to be entranced?

I've always enjoyed non-fiction and I'm holding on to that genre, for now. I'm progressing though a 500-page loan from my son Dan: *The Age of Wonder*, by British author and academic Richard Holmes. Holmes effortlessly blends science and biography; being married to novelist Rose Tremain might help him understand what it takes to create a fascinating story. Or maybe he helps her?

And speaking of good stories, historical fiction still welcomes me — Kate Grenville's *A Room Made of Leaves* was particularly enjoyable.

Before COVID-19, podcasts had moved in on my discretionary time. While I love their intimacy and the mind-blowing variety of subjects on offer, my experience is that the proliferation of home studios for broadcasting has reduced their quality. High-pitched voices or poor phone connections are not restful, whatever the topic. Mostly I settle on global affairs podcasts produced in purpose-built studios and, yes, discussions about books.

Each morning I scan several newspapers, national and international, on my iPad. I like the clear fonts, open spacing, short sentences. I'll read longer articles when I want to deep-dive into a topic. I don't buy print newspapers. I subscribe to *Griffith Review*, enjoying the way the essays connect with the zeitgeist. As a bonus, *GR* designers choose distinctive fonts that make reading pleasurable.

And poems. Good poems can be an exquisite blend of precision and soft focus. One can return to them again and again, finding even more to please the senses, the emotions and the mind. Poems are frequent visitors to my in-box. I look forward to receiving Kathryn Fry's latest poem — always a sensory feast whether she's connecting her reader with a plant, a tree, a bird or a landscape — often with subtle and surprising depth work under the surface. And from the other side of the world, a sensitively curated email arrives weekly from American poet James Crews. These chosen poems of gratitude and hope, together with his own, have taught me so much more about the art of paying attention in the moment. They have inspired and sustained me as I find my way through the weird terrain of these pandemic years.

I devote time and thought to encouraging my grandsons to read books, second-guessing what will engage them and tracking down titles. It's hard to compete against the giddy, fluoro-coloured world of video games. I alight on the idea of short stories — we can read one per visit, talk about what happened, catch difficult words in our 'improving comprehension' net. Perhaps short stories are part of the answer for me too.

What does it matter? I ask myself. Because I feel like I'm losing something, something that's been an integral part of my life. Because I feel that if I do let go of reading novels, I might miss out on learning something vital to my survival.

I'm a reader — that's part of my identity. Current affairs, essays, short stories, poems, historical fiction, even children's books that I 'road-test' for the boys are still in the mix. I'm not giving up after all, just reframing. I'm relieved to discover that, even if novels slide from my grasp, there is still an array of reading riches out there for me.

A sensible place

How many times had I leafed through the tray of pending papers on my desk? Searched the hanging file labelled 'Warranty' in the filing cabinet? Combed through the folders in 'the obvious drawer', the one with instruction manuals for our most-used electrical devices? I even put on disposable gloves and sorted through two bags of office waste from the garbage bin. My efforts were hopeless; the papers had disappeared.

A couple of weeks earlier, Ken had bought the latest PlayStation for our grandsons to use at our house. I'd taken the manual and a couple of other documents to record details like username and password on them for future reference. Missing one item of information, I'd put the papers aside until I could add it, intending to file them in a safe, appropriate place.

When I'd obtained the missing information, I couldn't find the papers. It was not a life-and-death matter. The manual is available online and I had stored the receipts separately. Why then was this upsetting me? Ken couldn't help.

'You're in charge of filing,' he said. 'But it shows our life is getting totally out of control.'

I couldn't agree with his wild exaggeration, but I hated the way this trivial loss made me feel. I couldn't trust my common sense to put those papers somewhere logical, or my memory of what I'd done with them.

Going to bed that night, I invoked a dream from my subconscious. It had worked before; next day an insight would arrive, and my problem would be solved. This time though, nothing happened.

After breakfast next morning, I decided to go through all the same old possible places once more, carefully. Thoroughly. I couldn't think of any new places to add to the list. I read somewhere that misplacing the car keys can happen to anyone, but putting things in inappropriate places — like the frying pan in the refrigerator — is definitely something to worry about. I wasn't going there.

The last place I searched was 'the obvious drawer'. This time, I delved well beneath the surface folders and there they were. Pristine in a plastic sleeve, my neatest handwriting on the top page, those papers seemed almost smug. Found at last! I rushed to show Ken, who was only mildly surprised and pleased.

Well, I'd put them in a sensible place. And I remembered that I could have put them there, in 'the obvious drawer'. I've passed on those two points. But I'd failed to search that drawer carefully enough. I'd assumed that they'd be close to the top. Now who on earth had been rummaging in that drawer, so that those particular papers had become buried?

It's tenuous, holding on to our capabilities as we age. And frightening — as we feel our fragile hold slipping, look around in alarm, try to keep our bearings in a slippery world. That hummingbird comes to mind again.

Are our lives ever under control, or is this just an illusion? I felt some small comfort, writing in the missing detail, scanning the papers, and filing them under 'Warranty'. If only life was that simple. But for now, it will do.

Faith in fluidity

It might sound depressing but it's not. We'd been binge-viewing movies about dementia over recent months — revisiting ones enjoyed before such as *Still Alice*, *Iris* and *Away from Her*; discovering the Korean gems *A Moment to Remember* and *Poetry*, as well as watching out for anything new. When *Supernova* arrived on our television screen, a whole different level of experience awaited.

Every film about this terrible disease is about love, in some way or other. The love that *Supernova* concerns itself with is between two men, Sam and Tusker, who have been together for decades. Tusker has early-onset dementia and is aware he is on a precipice. As they set off on a road trip in their motorhome, Tusker dithering over a map and Sam keeping calm at the wheel, I decide that Sam is the strong one. As the movie evolves, the opposite is revealed.

Tusker knows he is losing everything that has made him what he is, the ability to comprehend the world around him, to recognise the face and know the name of the man he loves. Yet he finds courage to engage with these losses, and plan for them in a way Sam will struggle to understand.

What is also revealed is that these two men will never stop loving each other. 'And it's testament to the performances given by Colin Firth and Stanley Tucci that we believe this *to our core*,' writes film critic Brian Tallerico, writing for *RogerEbert.com*. To say that we are witness to a truly loving relationship is totally inadequate — but we are — and we learn this mainly through their silences. 'They feel like people who know each other's body language; people who can sense change and emotional unrest in one another in ways that no one else can,' explains Tallerico.

Our preoccupation with dementia movies didn't spring out of nowhere. It's now almost a year since the multiple assaults on Ken's brain — a tumour, bleeding, surgerys and radiation therapy. Mild cognitive impairment has been the result and we've been observing subtle changes.

When Ken and I met in 2003, his mother had not long been admitted to a nursing home in Melbourne. By then aged 82, she was unable to speak or recognise family or friends. Her dementia symptoms became undeniable in 1994 when she was 75, but their seriousness suggested she'd been deteriorating for some years before. The coincidence of their ages, 75, when momentous things happened to mother and son, worried Ken. I, too, have been concerned about and conscious of my own cognitive fluctuations.

Ken sought out a geriatrician who gave him a thorough assessment. He learned that having had a tertiary education and been an engineer, he possessed cognitive reserves that would stand him in good stead. However, because of his craniotomies, he's at greater risk of an underlying dementing process.

As I think about how my relationship with Ken is shifting with the weight of our changing circumstances, I return to Tusker and Sam. In their relationship, there was still bickering, misunderstanding, denial of reality and attempts to influence and control one another. Just as in many long-term partnerships, ours too. But it was the experience of being drawn into that world of deep mutual empathy that stayed with me for days. It was remarkable. Something to be savoured, not easily absorbed by the superficial chatter and anxieties of everyday life.

In her classic *Gift from the Sea*, American aviator and author Anne Morrow Lindbergh writes that when one loves someone, it is impossible to love them in the same way, every moment of every day. Yet that is what many of us expect of ourselves, and of others. She urges us to have more faith in the ebb and flow of life, of love, of relationships. While we want permanence and continuity, Lindbergh says that the only continuity we can really be sure of is in growth, and in fluidity.

It's been a privilege for me, seeing faith in fluidity, in the ebb and flow, emerge during that film. Like walking into the sea, finding myself suddenly out of my depth, thrusting my arm forward, fingertips pointed, into the memory of swimming.

CHAPTER SIX

Sifting

On return

It had taken me days to work out how I felt about our journey to the north-west of NSW to visit the remains of my extended family there: a sister, a brother and his wife.

Ken and I had traversed a landscape that can be stripped bare in drought, torched by fire, drowned in floods or squandered in the abandon of too much grass. A landscape that shaped my growing up, a landscape that, at the mercy of something larger, promises nothing and forgives no one.

Late autumn 2021, tall pasture grasses jostle against the road verge. Water laps shallow lagoons and brims dams. Abundance is the word.

The trip divides itself in two: first, the Hunter Valley. The highway busy with mine-workers, school buses, scurrying mums and dads. Brutalist open-cut coalmines, dwarfing the modesty of roadside farmhouses, shocking the traveller as polished rock dazzles through trees. The towns of Muswellbrook, Singleton and Scone are alive and at work.

Beyond Tamworth, a sprawling regional centre, things begin to change. The soil turns a pale grey, leached of its nutritional value. The eucalypts, which my father called ironbarks, are ragged. In the small towns and villages we pass through, it seems there are not enough customers to sustain businesses, not enough staff to make consistently good-quality coffee or food for travellers keen to stop.

The owners of cafes and pubs along the way are wary of us, pointing sharply to the QR code we must scan. We're strangers, even though we bring welcome dollars. In Bingara, our destination, the Vodaphone service on my mobile provides only an SOS connection.

Joining my sister Jan and sister-in-law Lori for coffee, I struggle with the unfamiliarity of Ken's phone (which should work for a QR code) under the eye of the pub owner. Warning of dire fines for non-compliance, she signs me in.

When we visit my brother John, confined to his bed for the past 18 months with Parkinson's, Warialda high care staff are welcoming. In the lounge area, surrounded by residents, talk is of our long trip and past journeys John remembers. A care worker moves our little group to a quiet alcove and my brother falls asleep. At lunchtime Lori spoons food into his mouth but his eyes don't open. After two hours we leave, feeling desolate.

There are several places in Bingara where we can go for our evening meal. The first night in the Bingara RSL, Sunday, Ken comes close to collapse just as we reach our table. I order in haste and make a poor choice.

When we decide to give the club another chance on Monday night, it's in total darkness. We do the rounds; we hadn't known that most venues would be closed that night.

Despite many family kindnesses, we use all our back-up food: homemade soup, eggs, even baked beans. There's a particular loneliness about a country town at night, when only Telstra workers and those in need of a poker machine or a beer venture out.

I am overwhelmed by the sense that parts of rural Australia like this are being left behind. Expensive groceries, scarce medical services, ageing populations, not enough young people to provide essential services and labour. Lori has been waiting weeks for the only electrician in town to take the dying battery out of her smoke alarm. How she's tolerated the intermittent chirruping, I'll never know.

Jan loves her home of the past 50 years, 15 minutes drive from town. She's embedded in a strong community of mainly older women friends. She'll continue giving to others for as long as she is able, then it will be up to a younger generation to help her.

At home, unpacking slowly, I reflect on how challenging this trip has been. Not only for Ken who has been the driver in less than perfect health, needing to keep focused for endless kilometres, but also for me.

The practical matters of planning, packing, and navigating my immediate physical environment has consumed more energy than I'd expected. But it was the emotional impact of seeing family members at critical junctures of their lives that continued to reverberate after I returned home.

Throughout my life, I've regularly travelled long distances to renew my connections with loved ones. This time, as I immersed myself in their lives, I found myself feeling too intensely, being left raw and exposed.

Once home, I seek my own singular ways of counteracting that which has unsteadied me. Ken and I share our thoughts, revisiting them from different perspectives. The familiar ritual of unpacking and placing things back where they belong is balm for the soul. I sit at my computer and write, offering myself to the rhythm of my writing voice.

Mid-morning on Mother's Day, I hear a hustle at the front gate. Zeus and Cass burst into the house, trailed by their mum who is laden with carry-bags. Faces alight with smiles and anticipation, the boys throw their arms wide. Every sombre thought is sent scampering, chased by warmth and hugs.

A deeper truth

This is probably a surprise to those who know me, but sometimes I find it hard to articulate what I want to say, especially if feelings are involved. As a child I was very shy; visitors to our country home were rare and I remember running to hide under my bed when a strange car drew up at our gate. I was unschooled in the art of polite conversation.

In my first year at secondary school a teacher informed my mother that she thought I was a slow learner because it took me so long to find the words to express myself. Even now I sometimes find small talk challenging.

In adolescence I went through a stage of believing one had always to be honest and speak the truth. This struck others as being blunt or tactless: it was. My mother was devastated once, when returning home for university holidays, I told her how tired she looked. Back then, for me the truth always trumped diplomacy or dissembling. I wanted to hear the truth — why wouldn't others?

Over time I learned that 'saying it how it is' isn't inherently virtuous and can be hurtful. I've learned to be more sensitive to other people's feelings.

Unearthing my own feelings remains hard for me. Saying goodbye to Ken in the early morning stillness on yet another trip to hospital, I felt fear grab at my throat. How many more times would we do this, me seeing him off to do battle with a very clever enemy, one capable of a million disguises? I wanted to say something meaningful to him, intimate. Instead, I waved and, in silence, watched him disappear inside the taxicab.

'Not knowing what we have to say and having nothing to say are not the same thing,' Martin Bloch says in Alex Miller's novel *The Passage of Love*. 'We find out what we have to say when we attempt to say it. We think we want to say one thing, then in the attempt to say it we find there is a deeper and clearer truth waiting for us just below the surface of our first thought.'

Bloch is referring to writing but his words apply equally to voice. It's not that I have nothing to say; it's that what I have to say is deep in the subconscious. There's no time in the rapid interplay of everyday conversation to haul it to the surface and understand it, let alone express it. That's why it's easier for me to write than speak about things that are important to me — it gives me time to think and, if I am lucky, occasionally uncover that 'deeper and clearer truth'.

Maybe it is why most of us speak in superficialities — the first thoughts that come off the top of our heads. It's easiest. Who wants deep and meaningful anyway — there's a time and place for such discourse, to be chosen with care.

Feelings are becoming cheap fodder for the media. Journalists are sent 'into the field' — the scene of flood, fire, betrayal, murder — to find anyone, even a bystander, who can say how they feel. These informants satisfy by pulling up words like *angry, hurt, confused, devastated* . . . sometimes *thrilled, excited*. 'How excited are you about the win?' a breathless interviewer will ask a sporting fan. 'Oh, *incredibly*' is the reply. Is this news?

Getting in touch with our authentic feelings — not manufactured ones — can be the work of a lifetime for people like me who tend to view the world through a prism of rationality. I trust calm logic more than the feelings and emotions that threaten to destabilise me with their turmoil. Yet I have learned what a powerful role our emotions play in our decision-making, often directing from a very back seat, demolishing logical analysis in one sweep. A couple of my long-past relationship choices are cases in point. Looking back, I know now that it was my emotional self, hungry and demanding but voiceless, that powered those decisions.

During the late 1980s, I was drawn to the human-potential movement and attended workshops by the American author and philosopher Dr Jean Houston. Her blending of cross-cultural, mythic and spiritual teachings nourished me. That marked the beginning of my work over decades to bring my emotional and creative selves out of hiding and give them a voice.

Like the mythological Greek hero Odysseus and his journey of many vicissitudes from Troy to his Ithaca home, mine too is taking its time: In 'Ithaca', Greek poet C. P. Cavafy counsels:

> Always keep Ithaca fixed in your mind.
> To arrive there is your ultimate goal.
> But do not hurry the voyage at all.
> It is better to let it last for long years,

and even to anchor at the isle when you are old,
rich with all you have gained on the way,
not expecting that Ithaca will offer you riches.

Vanishing act

Writing short posts for my *Morning Pages* blog replaced my practice of keeping a journal. I was writing in more depth, allowing events and feelings to be a catalyst for a different way of understanding experiences of my daily life. My focus was on what was close, domestic — small, even — but the effect was transformative. I'd learned how to do something new, and I wanted to keep doing it.

Journal writing had become a way of holding on to my identity, my sense of self, and my memories. It was as if writing made things real. I kept journals to capture important passages in my life, pin them to the page, so I wouldn't forget. I have boxes and boxes of them, the handwriting becoming less legible as the years pass.

Some I converted to typed summaries and drew on for a memoir of my near-decade living on the far north coast of NSW, titled *Moving North: The Long Way Home*. The draft was several years in the writing. When I was satisfied, it was placed in a computer file labelled Unpublished. There it remained, for another few years.

My remarriage and move north in 2003 happened suddenly; it was far harder to adjust to the change than I'd imagined. I felt torn between my new life and partner, and my family. The excruciating exacerbations of MS I experienced were aggravated by stress and the hot, humid climate. I persisted in writing the memoir as therapy, a way of understanding what I was going through.

I chose the year 2021 to place the draft memoir in the hands of a Sydney editor, Shelley Kenigsberg. Daily life would be constrained by the pandemic so I would have time and emotional space to take the manuscript to the next level of development. I'd also gain some sense of whether memoir writing was something I could do.

In all, I've had four books published — one in the broad self-help genre, two social histories and one family history. I know what is involved in bringing a substantial written work into form and to market. I had no interest in taking the manuscript of that deeply personal memoir to a wider audience. It had another function.

As I worked through each paragraph, responding to my editor's perceptive suggestions, revisiting events and emotions, I discovered something surprising. The sense of loss that had permeated much of my time on the far north coast had evaporated. It was as if it had all happened to someone else.

Australian author Alex Miller explains in his book *The Simplest Words: A Storyteller's Journey* that he does not tell a story to get to the end but to find its centre, the dilemma at its heart. I knew that in writing that memoir, I'd have to deep-dive below the surface turbulence, to find its centre. That's what I sought to do.

Was the process of writing in the end therapeutic? My friend Cecile Yazbek, herself a memoirist, offered a perspective from a different angle: 'Our writing, exploring wounds and scars, could be overwhelming. Instead, word by word, *we lay a pathway.'*

Years of journal writing served to clarify my thoughts and provide a safety valve for my feelings. Writing that memoir *was* laying a pathway. Eventually, through that process, finding the heart of my dilemma and in the passage of time, healing did happen. The memoir had served its purpose.

I'm not ready to bin my boxes of old journals just yet. I don't know if there's raw material sitting there that can be used for fresh alchemical purposes. If there is, I'm not sure if I have the stamina to tackle that work. Nor am I sure I can repeat the magic. I'll not stop writing; that much I know.

Movement in stillness

The winter solstice on Monday 21 June 2021 was the shortest day of the year, a marker of the deepest point in winter, after which the nights become shorter and the days brighter. For me it was a watershed, a time of sifting, settling, and resolving.

It's one of the most powerful points of the year as the axis of the earth pauses, shifts and moves in the opposite direction. 'For three days around the solstice we experience the spiritual power of the standstill point and the shift of direction,' writes Chloe Rain, founder of the blog *Explore Deeply*. She suggests the winter solstice can be a metaphor for a pause to look within and take stock of our lives, even changing direction with intent.

When a cyst began growing on my lower eyelid, I decided to wait and see what it would do. Ken and I set off on a much-postponed mini-break up the coast. On return, the cyst had grown, but my regular GP was fully booked for 10 days. With a stroke of luck, I seized a cancellation that had popped up on the schedule of a new doctor he'd recommended if he wasn't available. She was calm and measured, removing the cyst, and offering a slightly different perspective on a couple of bothersome issues I'd been tolerating.

Next, I visited the MS Clinic at John Hunter Hospital for an annual review of my MS. Dr M, a young neurologist whom I'd met before, gave me a thorough assessment. She was pleased that I'd had no serious exacerbations for three or more years and that going to the gym twice weekly was obviously helping to build my muscle strength.

A new drug, Siponimod, had recently been approved for use in patients with secondary MS and, most importantly, was available, and financially accessible, under the Pharmaceutical Benefits Scheme. I'd come prepared to discuss this and thought it may be offered to me. Privately, I'd reached the conclusion that I wouldn't risk disturbing the stability I'd achieved and expose myself to increased vulnerability to infections.

For Dr M, it seemed a question barely worth considering. 'We've got about 40 patients on it,' she explained. 'And so far, it's showing benefits mainly for those whose disease is active.' After a moment, she went on.

'Yours isn't active, now. But MS can spring up suddenly, even after a long period of quiet. If that happens for you, we've now got something to offer.' Her voice was resonant with warning.

'In the meantime,' Dr M said, 'we can get another MRI done. You've not had one for three years, so it's time.'

Stability was the watchword for Ken too; he'd just completed his three-monthly rounds of surveillance scans and specialist appointments. Everyone was pleased. He's less well than I am but manages to do the things that are most important to him. That's his own self-care and medical appointments, and support for me and for our grandsons here in Newcastle. As the boys grow up, our role is changing but not lessening, as they each have special educational needs. Fatigue means Ken has had to let go of the many handyman jobs he used to do; he can't drive long distances; he struggles sometimes to keep on track and complete all the elements of a task he's embarked on. But he is taking on more household chores.

At last our home help is running smoothly: a cleaner comes once a fortnight but only for two hours. I do everything he doesn't, but I have a routine and I'm getting quicker. I've found an energetic young woman to help maintain our courtyards and small front garden. I arrange an online delivery of staple groceries once every six weeks. I've simplified our meals and cook. All our heavy crockery has been replaced by lightweight Corelle. Having systems in place is part of minimising our risks. We're both aware of how quickly things can fall apart.

At this time of shifting energies, there's a sense of having moved into a place of equilibrium. As the sun stood still at the time of solstice, I thought of my good fortune. While some things have been resolved and concluded, other, different pathways have been revealed. Things are not as they once were. Like the tremble of first light on calm water, even in stillness movement is inevitable.

A step ahead

It wasn't 'shabby chic', just 'shabby', the light-commercial neighbourhood we moved into in 2012. But even then, signs of rejuvenation were beginning to appear — accounting offices replacing a car sales yard; fresh decals on the solicitor's expansive glass frontage; a stylish fit-out for the beautician.

COVID-19 took its toll on Newcastle, but the power of renewal was stronger. In my suburb, Hamilton, a handful of businesses closed but it was surprising during 2021 to see the flush of new owners buying into cafes and hotels with fresh ideas. Perhaps landlords were becoming a little more realistic in the rents they were asking, but the supply of people keen to 'have a go' seemed strong. The Hamilton Business Association reported 32 new businesses moving here in the past 12 months, many offering eating-out experiences I'd yet to try.

The City of Newcastle had responded to a submission I'd made five years previously asking for kerb ramps to be installed along footpaths near my home. How much easier and safer these new ramps made it for me, pushing my walker or riding my mobility scooter. And after years of community consultation, the City fast-tracked plans to redevelop Hamilton's small central plaza into an attractive flexible-use space. Contemporary art structures and etchings, on which I'd advised, celebrate the suburb's history and heritage.

As Melbourne and other cities struggle to reimagine their central business districts, Newcastle has enjoyed a head start. With the closure of the

BHP steelworks in 1999, crowds surging along Newcastle city streets on paydays became a distant memory even for ageing Novocastrians, to be marvelled at only in sepia photographs on the Lost Newcastle Facebook page.

The central area of Newcastle used to remind me of a person who had shrunk inside their clothes, clothes that now hung loose, baggy, far too big. Unused buildings were everywhere, many once beautiful, caught in a time warp of a bygone era when there were simply many more people.

Now a makeover is underway. The grand dame that was Newcastle is getting a totally new wardrobe, the latest fashion — and if the fit is not yet perfect, it is better. And the COVID-induced flight to the regions is fortuitous timing for our city.

Today what was once the CBD is a cacophony of building works, multi-storey buildings in progress wherever one looks. Original facades are retained where feasible, often in response to community pressure. While many commercial offices still line the foreshore of the Hunter River, it is no longer a CBD but a 'lifestyle precinct'. Residents of the proliferating apartment buildings step out to cafes, bars, hotels, galleries, markets, speciality shops, foreshore parklands and the beach. The City of Newcastle is spending millions transforming heritage sites such as The (Railway) Station and upgrading city and coastal infrastructure — plazas and parks, baths and ocean pools, walkways and playgrounds. Newcastle is becoming a very liveable city.

On the mornings I go to the gym, Ken roams far afield, discovering new building works and enjoying what must be world-class views of the industrious river port and city beaches. A couple of my classmates take this walk from their homes, each time seeing it with fresh eyes and having something to share on arrival.

A business owner in the city centre, where disruption is in full swing, told me: 'We can see the future; it looks great. We've survived the worst, while the whole place was just dying. Now there's commitment, and we'll make it.'

She went on to say she'd already come to know residents from the surrounding apartments. 'People have moved here from everywhere,' she said. 'I've met some lovely people. They are so glad to be here, and don't complain that everything is still a massive construction site.'

Ken takes a more pessimistic view. With his engineer's mindset, he iterates everything not planned for, things that could go wrong, unintended consequences of such rapid, intense development, especially of high-rise apartments.

Back home, the test of the gentrification of my immediate locality is an empty building on our street corner. Once part of an 1870s structure that stretched the whole block, it was the popular Blatchford's Bakery until the 1989 earthquake, ending its days as a rental property that frequently changed tenants. When would it be demolished, or even transformed? A development application to build — yes, a boutique apartment block — had been lodged a couple of years ago. But the project seemed to have stalled.

Then one day, as I pushed my walker along the street, I saw a small sign stuck in the soil against the building. It was the logo and name of the builder engaged for the project. Excited, I shared the news with Ken on my return. He grumbled about the pressure the works would add to our tiny street; even the new kerb ramp there was likely to be sacrificed.

There's no sign of anything starting yet. But my spirits lift when I see another business start-up or land cleared for a new building where one was derelict and unloved before. Things might not always work out as planned, but I choose to listen to the message. It's one of hope — of someone making a commitment to the place, a promise of renewal, revitalisation. It's someone investing in our city, creating a better future for our children, grandchildren, and theirs.

A tumultuous decade

It has been a mammoth job, trawling through over 30 years of personal journals and extracting memorable events and experiences for a digital record. During the pandemic, it was something I could always pick up, like knitting, when I didn't know what else to do. And sure enough, eventually it was finished.

Throughout this process, I fell under a spell. This had been my life, yet it seemed distant and unreal, as if it belonged to someone else.

It was reading over the life-changing events of the 1990s that impressed themselves most powerfully on my psyche. The breakdown of my marriage and coparenting our three teenage children; walking away from the security of a public service job to establish my own business; the publication of my first book.

Daily meditation was part of my life over those years, along with yoga. I immersed myself in mastering NLP (neurolinguistic programming), a form of psychotherapy somewhat like cognitive behavioural therapy. I learned empowering ways of thinking to help me set boundaries, respond resourcefully to criticism, or resolve internal conflicts. Knowing how to reframe difficult situations and my own less productive behaviours and attitudes stands me in good stead even today. As my skills and confidence grew, my consciousness changed too. This flowed through to the way I communicated with people in my client organisations, assisting them to achieve the outcomes they wanted.

Meanwhile, I'd begun a long-distance relationship with Richard, lasting almost six years. I criss-crossed the continent for work, as he did; we became expert at creating opportunities to see and do things that brought both pleasure and respite to our hectic lives.

That tumultuous decade was, for me, transformative. Reliving those years through my journals, I was filled with envy. I carried that feeling around for days, more than a week. Where has my life gone? Can I get it back? What am I now, a shadow?

Other questions surface. Confronting the details of a relentless work schedule, the pressures I put myself under, I wonder: Was I mad? *How* did I do it? *Why* did I do it?

The consequences were revealed in 1997, when after a series of intractable infections, I was diagnosed with MS. Richard flew to Sydney immediately to be with me.

I didn't stop for long: fresh out of five days of infusions with anti-inflammatory medication, I was off again, this time to the USA. 'Go!' urged my neurologist. 'Go!'

Over time, I learned to pace myself, but a pattern of 'boom and bust' is clear in my journals. Periods of intense work, travel and recreation, followed by collapse from exhaustion. It seems I willingly paid the price.

English blogger and writer Josie George lives with a chronic health condition that has never been satisfactorily diagnosed. The insights she shares on her blog, *Bimblings*, are at once simple and profound. In a post titled 'Excavation', she writes about wiping dust from her bedroom cabinet, chopping a tomato, feeling pain in her stomach, hanging up the t-shirt her boy will wear tomorrow: these things are living. Rushing through them 'thoughtlessly, panicked, bitter, hungry for more . . . is to rush through time as if it were nothing . . . ' she says. These moments are her life.

Such things are my life, too. I'm glad I can look back on the 1990s as a time when I had the courage to upend my life and take it in a completely different direction. Just as I sped up then, I slow down now. Josie George concludes:

> What a surprise it is: I have slowed down and I did not drown. My life is imperfect, hard, uncertain, but it is here, it is happening in my body and my body is alive, and to notice it again feels like baptism. Outside, the world races ahead and leaves me behind, but for the first time in a long time, I don't think I mind.

Heart circle

It popped onto my screen, the top result of a desultory Google search. An obituary notice, his name at the top. Next line: 'Died suddenly'.

I'd been transcribing events from my 1998 journal, and Richard had been a constant presence in those pages. A few days before finding the notice, I'd emailed him. The address was 20 years old, so unlikely to still be active. I kept my message brief. No reply came to my email, but I was not surprised.

I'm not sure what made me type his name into the Google search bar, but it doesn't matter. Clearly, he was on my mind.

Richard had been one of the most influential people in my life. We'd met through my health consulting work and instantly sparked off each other. Slightly younger than me, he consumed sports — tennis, skiing, golf, cycling — and his passion, birds. He was fit and healthy, living life to the full every minute of every day.

In those heady days, we both travelled often. I was divorced, my children in their adolescence. They had a father, much loved, and didn't need another, even at a distance. That suited both of us. When possible, we synchronised our travel commitments or made opportunities to do things together in interesting places. Our relationship provided excitement and comfort in equal measure.

To be honest, there was angst as well.

Stunned by my discovery of Richard's death, I spent the day in a daze. His father had been diagnosed with dementia at a relatively young age and I'd always assumed that this would be Richard's fate. What did 'died suddenly' mean? A fatal stroke, an aneurysm, a heart attack? I didn't want to know.

I shared my feelings with Ken and with my lifelong friend Leigh Toop, a Canberra artist. I told her I'd always felt secure in the knowledge that Richard was 'out there, somewhere', even though we'd not spoken for almost two decades. That I could phone him, and he would be there for me at once, attentive, caring, ready to listen and advise. No matter that our relationship had ended back in 1999, that I'd remarried in late 2003 and declined his wish that we keep in touch.

Leigh responded with empathy and affection borne of long years knowing each other. 'Even though 20+ years have passed since your relationship came to an end,' she emailed, 'at another level I don't feel relationships ever end. There is always unfinished or unexpressed business . . . gratitude, disappointment, forgiveness, a sense of betrayal, or whatever.'

I have trouble accepting that the vibrant, curious, energetic man with whom I'd shared a few years of my life was gone, no more, dead. Then I recalled his words to me after one visit in 1998, even as our relationship was almost over: 'If I had only two such experiences a year,' he'd said, 'I'd think myself lucky.'

We'd been lucky, many times over.

Finding meaning

Mid-winter, July 2021, the month of my birth. Across NSW, Victoria and South Australia more than half the population of our nation was in lockdown. The Delta strain of COVID-19 was leading experts on a crazy guessing game. And as the wreckers demolished the 150-year-old building on my street corner, screeches, thuds and subterranean shudders traumatised our quiet home. My footings, like the world around me, felt shaky and precarious.

In his aged care facility, my immobile brother had been locked in a battle for his life. He'd emerged from an onslaught of infections the victor — barely. Through it all, I moved back and forth to my daughter's house, finding surprising respite in passing hours with her boys in simple school holiday activities.

When I began writing and blogging again a year earlier, in June 2020, it was a desperate lurch for solid ground. Ken's melanoma had spread to his brain; I'd had emergency eye surgery. The COVID-19 pandemic had been named and we were enduring a 90-day period of restrictions on our movements. Everything seemed to be closing in on us. I needed to save myself, to survive the present and prepare for what lay ahead.

The opening post in the *Morning Pages* blog that emerged on 6 July 2020 summoned me — and my readers — to do what made us joyous. But in these uncertain and terrible times, I asked myself, is the pursuit of joy heartless, an extravagance we can't afford?

Over the writing months that followed, my musings morphed into something else. Whatever the subject, every post seemed, at its heart, to be about finding meaning. The process of writing was itself an act of mindfulness, of pausing to pay attention to whatever had settled before me. And like an archaeologist patiently paring debris clinging to a precious object, I excavated meaning.

As I wrote and shared my discoveries with a cluster of invited readers, my insights were deepened by theirs. I have felt comforted, both by the kernels of meaning I was uncovering in my experiences, and the resonances my words found in their lived experience.

Going deeper, I discovered something remarkable, especially for someone like me who places a high value on endurance. I found not just meaning, but the comfort of meaning.

CHAPTER SEVEN

Things Fall Apart

Qué pasa?

'What's happening? How are things? What's up?' *Qué pasa?* I learned this popular multi-purpose greeting on our travels in Spain, though I didn't always grasp the fine details of the answer, delivered in rapid-fire Spanish. For days *Qué pasa?* has been hovering in my consciousness; I've been feeling the need to make a list, but things don't stop happening.

On Thursday 5 August 2021, Newcastle and LGAs north and south were ordered into lockdown. It followed Greater Sydney's, which began on 26 June. It was anticipated here for weeks; our city had been on edge wondering how on earth we'd escaped so far. When the answer came, I was about to leave for an appointment. The audiologist's usually calm office was vibrating with the radio news of the immediate lockdown, the receptionist already contacting clients to cancel appointments.

I'd planned to stop at the pharmacy on my way home; now I added Sanderson Meats. A queue extended out the door of Graham's small shop, an unusual sight. Inside, I found him alone behind the counter, valiantly serving amid whole chunks of lamb, beef and a kind of controlled chaos.

It was easy to cancel my personal commitments. Rozlyn my hairdresser was the first to phone — yes, Bella Mia was required to close. So was the gym. A text message arrived from Zeus's dad, cancelling a family birthday dinner for our grandson. More complicated negotiations followed for the face-to-face English tutorials I'd recently arranged for him, and the logistics that hinged on them. Because Vino was an essential worker, both her boys would attend school for three days each week and have home learning when their mother was home. On the first day of the lockdown, Vino busied herself setting up computers and passwords, reporting, with relief, that the boys' school appeared to have relaxed their expectations somewhat compared to the previous year.

What else had been happening? I'd turned 76 and Ken had given me his favoured gift, technology. A new iPhone and iPad arrived, and while he offered to do the initial start-up, I would be doing everything else. That included installing the apps, making sure everything mirrored my old devices and entering numerous passwords. Ken, never one to mince words, declared, 'You're going to have to do this yourself when I'm dead.'

Then he tackled our tax returns. Most of the forms are pre-filled these days but some choices are left for us. Ken completed his, then urged me to do mine, though I'm always jittery at the thought of handling paperwork relating to my financial and legal affairs. Now, despite last-minute hitches, it's done, successfully lodged with the ATO. All I must do next year is remember how to manage that curve ball my health insurance threw at me. Whether Ken is still here or not.

Another task hanging over me for months but being deferred was modernising my *Hidden Hamilton* blog. I'm proud that in 2013 I mastered blogging myself, without any help from Ken. While it's been virtually untouched by me for over three years, it remains in demand. Recent initiatives by the City of Newcastle and Hamilton Business Association stimulated interest in

Hamilton's history and this flowed through to my blog and book sales.

I had to get professional help but didn't know where to turn. I was wary of the cost for what was, essentially, a volunteer project. Then, in a mind flash, I realised my friend and colleague Jacq Hackett might help. In no time I was connected to her virtual assistant, Sharyn Munro — a talented Brisbane woman who could turn her hand to any research, administrative or technology task. In a small coincidence, she'd once lived in a street near us while at Newcastle TAFE; in another, she found my contact details already in her database. Apparently, I'd engaged her 15 or more years ago when I was consulting, and she was starting her new business.

As we worked on my blog through the weeks, Sharyn gave it a fresh new look, and did sophisticated things that made the blog easier to navigate. I realised I could make many necessary changes myself. But most interesting of all was the discovery of what it was like to have someone to simply 'hold my hand', someone who could get me out of trouble if I ventured too far into the treacherous terrain of cyberspace.

Settling into the seclusion of lockdown, I wondered how we in NSW had endured a 90-day lockdown the previous year. The plans our Prime Minister came up with to help us 'live with the virus' included no mention of contingency, as if the Delta variant of COVID-19 was the worst we could expect.

Qué pasa? A lot, actually. I walked up to my fears, gained new skills and confidence. Small in the scheme of things, I know, but something told me we were going to need every bit of courage and flexibility for what lay ahead.

Something, or nothing

They roll around every three months without fail, a series of scans and medical appointments monitoring the melanoma my husband lives with. This time he has been muttering about things not being 'quite right'.

The first of the series is a PET scan. Ken is now able to once again drive himself to the imaging centre. Yesterday, however, a small errand to a nearby suburb felt a challenge for him and he asked me to come with him. Ever since the brain surgery over a year ago, he's experienced disorientation when moving from sitting to standing. It passes, but he takes a minute or two to steady himself and feel secure enough to move off.

'That's not getting any better,' he tells me. 'In fact, I think it's getting worse.'

He reports something similar in transitioning from screen-focused computer work to standing and looking around; his vision is affected. No medical specialist, optometrist, physiotherapist or exercise physiologist can shed light on this.

'It's neurological' is the catch-all explanation.

When a large parcel was delivered recently, he carried it inside and began unpacking. We often complain about the difficulty of breaking into packaging these days, from the smallest product like batteries to the larger ones, like this stick vacuum cleaner. Ken was bending over slightly, wrestling the big box. Eventually, after great effort, he succeeded in extricating the appliance. Next, he sat down with a book of instructions written in idiosyncratic English in minuscule font.

The vacuum cleaner was complicated, and it took Ken some time to assemble it. It would have been hard for me because I was never much good at such things. Not so Ken. Like my brother John, who was skilled at mechanics — Ken could fix anything. This time, the task challenged and distressed him.

I was reminded of a story my sister-in-law told me. One day on the farm, John set off to the shed to do a minor repair. He seemed to be gone a long time; when he returned eventually, he was confused and upset. He told her he hadn't been able to do the task. He'd forgotten the process.

Recently, Ken has helped me solve a couple of computer problems. Or rather, he solved them when I had given up. Watching him, though, he seemed slower, less sure than usual. He urged me to be patient with him. He'd not forgotten the process, yet, but I feared for him.

My brother went on to be diagnosed with Lewy body dementia, and advanced Parkinson's disease. Both conditions 'neurological'.

Ken and I talk frankly about the changes affecting him. Things are happening for me, too; I draw on all my available resources to manage and my glitches arise mainly from ignoring the maxim 'less haste, more care'. When, I wonder, will the line be crossed when these explanations don't suffice?

'I will really worry,' Ken tells me, 'when I go down the street to the baker, get the bread, and forget my way home.'

So where was I?

'**Where's the homemade** muesli?' A plaintive cry drifted up the stairs. 'It's there, same place!' I called back. 'Look to the left'.

Ken was home, less than 48 hours after departing for brain surgery. It had been 'something', as he'd speculated. A small lesion previously noted in the right occipital lobe of his brain had grown and was thought to be a melanoma metastasis. He'd needed another craniotomy to remove it.

Now he was grappling with what seems to be the temporary loss of the left peripheral visual field, impinging on the visual cortex of the brain. To see what is there — a person, a car, a plate — he must remember to turn his head. He's learning.

Ken is a poor hospital patient. On discharge from ICU, he was wheeled into a two-bed ward of the private hospital. Its occupant was coughing constantly and listening to the races at full volume. The nurse explained that the man was hearing-impaired. 'Well, I can't cope with that noise,' said Ken, adamant. 'I want a private room.' Muttering about the hospital being full, the nurse went off to check. Ken got his single room.

Next morning I received a call from a different nurse, Linda. 'Ken thinks he's going home today,' she told me. 'He was up at 6 am looking for towels so he could have a shower. Patients don't shower until after breakfast!'

I pointed out that Ken's surgeon had told him he could go home this day, Thursday. 'It's early, though, isn't it, after brain surgery?' I queried.

'Definitely; I don't think he should go home. But he's determined.'

'I agree, but why don't you check with the surgeon?' I suggested. 'Ken will do whatever he says.'

Reassured, Linda went off. She phoned me back five minutes later.

'Yes, Dr F did tell him that,' she reported. 'He can go home if you can manage.'

If I can manage. I've heard that before. Hospitals are stressful, noisy places and Ken is super-sensitive to noise. During the night he'd gone into the corridor, searching for a sound he thought sounded like a staple gun. A nurse returned him promptly to his bed.

Once home, Ken discovered he'd lost his memory of the layout of the house. Heading for the bathroom, he found himself at the exit door to the garage. His short-term memory for where he'd put small items like lip salve or Panadol was disordered. He had forgotten the processes for making calls and sending messages on his phone. With single-minded determination, he set out to relearn.

Later, he spoke to his GP, who assured him this confusion was most likely a consequence of the anaesthetic and would soon resolve. It did, somewhat; Ken began to settle and grow calmer.

Home is more peaceful than hospital.

One day, Ken announced he was going to the baker to get the bread.

'I'd better come with you,' I replied, anxious.

'No, no, I'll be fine,' he said.

I let him go.

Within 15 minutes, he was back. He had not only remembered to buy the bread; he'd remembered the way home.

Secret weapon

It feels as though I'm draped with the weightiest of blankets, canvas even, a wet tent collapsed over me. My right leg struggles to respond; barely conscious, its messenger nerves are deadened. Movement is a deliberate act that must be thought, planned, then executed.

Fatigue. Its approach has been slow, imperceptible. It might have been the humidity, or that I've been unusually busy. Then, on a day when the skies opened and became indiscernible from the rain that poured out of them without ceasing, I recognised it. Its head above the parapet of my awareness, I realised I knew what it was, after all.

Over the past couple of years, I've been remarkably free of fatigue. It's one of the most common symptoms of MS. Being neurological, it doesn't respond to a good night's sleep like muscular tiredness does. I'm on a three-month regimen of injections of vitamin B12; that helps to some extent.

Something is different. In the evening, after Ken and I have enjoyed a movie, I haul myself out of the chair to take the elevator upstairs. I wish I could just drop straight into bed. The thought of undressing, washing my face, taking medications and performing other pre-bedtime rituals overwhelms me. I sit on the chair beside the bed, lean forward, begin to unlace my shoes, and unwrap my orthotic.

A coach once told me how to get motivated to build a fitness routine into one's daily life. 'In the morning, put on your sneakers, very first thing!' he says. 'Then you are on your way.'

That really does work. Grab hold of your sneakers, and you've broken through. At night, for me, it's the reverse. I just need to get started taking *off* my shoes, then the other tasks follow. My actions become almost automatic; it never occurs to me to skip part of the routine.

Mental conditioning and B12 injections are great but I need something more. I rummage in my medications drawer and find the bottle of Prednisone tablets. A corticosteroid with a range of side effects, oral Prednisone is the most powerful medication in my armoury, short of presenting myself at the hospital for an intravenous infusion. It is reputed to help reduce the inflammation associated with an MS exacerbation and calm an out-of-control immune system. I take the tablets for 14 days, phasing them down after the first three days to prevent withdrawal symptoms.

Usually I delay starting a course of Prednisone until I'm totally sure I'm having an exacerbation, but this deep fatigue is unmistakeable. Another reason for my reluctance to take corticosteroids is the way they disrupt my sleeping patterns. Early in the course when the dose is relatively high, I not only feel invigorated but could also stay up all night! That's not sustainable and I have limited ways of dealing with insomnia. A course of Prednisone is not something to be embarked upon lightly. There is some doubt now about whether the protocol recommended to me all those years ago by my Sydney neurologist is sufficient for a significant MS exacerbation. That's where an infusion comes in.

Within a few short days, I am feeling much better. At the gym, the exercise physiologist is surprised at the higher steps-per-minute I'm recording on the cross-trainer. She asks me what else I've been doing to achieve such good results, but I just smile and shake my head. We all need one — a secret weapon.

Who will listen to my dreams?

It's not unusual for both Ken and me to have strange dreams in the netherworld between the night's deep sleep and preparing to wake. Seated in the easy chair next to my bed, Ken tells his dream first, afraid he'll lose the details. Then I'll share mine. I've learned not to offer unsolicited analysis of the symbolism of Ken's dreams — it's enough to listen.

Ken's dream is a recurring one, but this morning it has an edge, and he seems disturbed. He describes being in a house, one he was very familiar with, and he thinks I was there. Walking around, he noticed a door he'd not seen before; going through, it opened into a whole new section of the house. Bedroom, bathroom, sitting area. 'It was very nice, and such a surprise,' he said. 'How come I'd missed it, all these years?' Knowing Ken, not noticing would have been unthinkable.

Because of Ken's engineering background, his dreams usually echo life situations where he's under pressure to fix something or solve a problem in real time. In his dreams he's trying to do a repair but can't find the correct part; he's travelling somewhere and gets lost because the directions are wrong. He becomes stressed and frustrated.

This time he feels confused and anxious. He doubts his grasp of reality. Were the extra rooms really there or were they an illusion? If they were there, what does that say about his usually excellent observation?

I decide to venture an interpretation, at my risk. 'Could the newly discovered rooms be an aspect of your future life that you are glimpsing for the first time? A place you are entering?'

I'm thinking of death, of course. Ken understands; there's no need for me to spell it out. I soften. 'Or perhaps what is being revealed are resources you didn't realise were available to you?'

He nods slowly.

'Remember how annoyed you get when you and I disagree — what colour something is, the order in which something happened,' I say. 'I don't really care who is right — it doesn't matter to me. But it is really important to you, because if you are proved wrong, you say it casts doubt on the accuracy of your perception or understanding.'

Ken agrees. 'That's a slippery slope; I feel as if my world is suddenly unstable, unreliable.'

'Then there are a few different ways of understanding your dream,' I conclude. 'But what is new is your confusion. That's not a good sign. Let's keep a watch on that.'

By now my own dream has dissipated, and I pull myself up and get out of bed. My chance to share will come another time. Indonesian-born American poet Li-Young Lee writes in his poem

'To Hold' about making the bed with his wife, aligning the sheets, the 'tug, fold, tuck' of the routine task. If he's lucky, he thinks, his wife will share a recent dream with him. Hovering at the edges of the poem is a foreshadowing of mortality, alongside an implication that worrying too much about loss and change in the future prevents us living in the present moment:

> So often, fear has led me
> to abandon what I know I must relinquish
> in time. But for the moment,
> I'll listen to her dream,
> and she to mine, our mutual hearing
> > calling
> more and more detail into the light
> of a joint and fragile keeping.

It's a fragile hold Ken and I have on each of our lives, we know. We've always been frank with each other, although there are tender areas in each of our psyches that call for care, like a bruise on the sole of one's foot caused by a sharp stone. Perhaps those sensitive spots are the hidden rooms in Ken's dream, yet to be explored and fully understood, allowed into consciousness at last.

A relationship like no other

'**I won't keep** carrying you,' I declared. 'I know you're not that heavy now, but if we continue like this, it will be a real drag. Something's got to change — starting today!'

I stepped off the scales, feeling resolution surge in my chest. Post-Christmas 2021, I'd put on almost two kilos in a month and I was annoyed with myself. Like other people, we'd had food left over from the festive season because the end-of-year COVID-19 outbreak had kept visitors close to home. Ken and I gradually consumed the excess, mindful of the use-by dates, enjoying the continuing small luxuries.

But our bodies are finely calibrated to energy in/energy out, mine especially because I am constrained in the 'energy out' category. I have a finite daily capacity, which, when expended, plunges me into exhaustion. Not so the 'energy in' — I'm not a big eater, but I love fresh summer fruits, creamy yoghurts and desserts, and crusty sourdough bread. All that, plus a glass of white wine in the courtyard's evening cool, is enough to destabilise my careful weight management system.

'Don't be too hard on yourself,' my inner voice says. 'Hardly indulgent — and you deserve a bit of pleasure after the year you've just endured.'

That's true. Yet it's also true that I need to despatch my two kilos because they will likely become three, even four, if I don't pay more attention to my eating. There they are again — those words, pay attention. I've not paid attention because my focus has been elsewhere.

Four weeks ago, in mid-December, restrictions were lifted in NSW at a dangerous time — cases of the Omicron variant began to escalate rapidly. Yet we were offered the reward of not just a real family Christmas, but the opportunity to dine, drink and party unhampered by masks, QR codes, density limits or social distancing. It was a confluence of all the elements for a perfect storm, resulting in a January deluge of tens of thousands of new cases.

Thousands of healthcare workers were on furlough due to contact with the virus, while those remaining were stressed and exhausted, at times beyond their ability to cope. Pictures of decimated supermarket shelves appeared on the evening news as workers and drivers critical to the supply chain fell ill or entered isolation.

'A strong society needs a strong economy,' proclaimed NSW Premier Dominic Perrottet. 'You can't run a healthy economy without healthy people,' retorted economist Professor Jim Stanford. Just days after NSW Health Minister Brad Hazzard warned that our state would reach 28,000 new cases by the end of January, more than 45,000 were reported on 8 January 2022. A hasty adjustment was made to the restrictions, but the situation was out of control.

Until a month earlier, I had known only one person who had contracted the virus, my niece in England. Now it was my son, his wife and one of their children in Sydney; my daughter and family members in Newcastle; a nephew and his wife; people who helped us; others whose names I'd lost track of. My daughter knew several who were suffering much more than she was; she's grateful to be triple vaccinated.

In this hiatus, holiday and childcare plans were upended and uncertainties proliferated. Distracted and preoccupied, I found it hard to settle. My addiction to the news returned. It was hard to make decisions, to determine how much risk was acceptable. The same amount of emotional energy could be expended on deciding whether to fly interstate to visit an ailing family member as to meet a friend for coffee in a local cafe. My friend Vicki emailed, 'Sometimes I'm OK with living the quiet life and other times I think I'll go mad!'

I'd cancelled everything I was planning for January — much-anticipated meetings with friends, a hair appointment, adjustments to my hearing aids, even my beloved gym. Seemingly trivial, such activities form the scaffolding of daily life. They hold us up.

It was harder not seeing my grandsons, but we innovated in cyberspace. And there was a big reason for my caution: Ken had begun receiving immunotherapy infusions. In November, just eight weeks after his second brain operation, a new metastasis of his melanoma was discovered in a lymph node. He was vulnerable to infection, and I didn't intend to take even the smallest risk of bringing COVID-19 into our home.

There was much talk about 'learning to live with COVID-19'. Having written about how I'm learning to live with MS, and Ken with melanoma, I reached for a more useful insight into this 'learning to live with . . .' concept. Is it something to do with a deep, primary relationship that is like no other — our relationship with our body?

That relationship is not an option. Except in death, we can't escape our body, though we can shape it to some extent. Its virtues and flaws go with us through our entire lives. Like every other real-life relationship, it supports and nurtures us, disappoints us, even makes us angry sometimes. But we're together for the span of our natural lives, and we have a responsibility to that relationship.

What 'living with . . .' has taught me is to ask my body questions, listen to it, and to take care of it. When next I step on the scales, I won't be upbraiding myself. I'll be paying closer attention to my body: taking note of what it tells me and acting in the best interests of us both. After all, we still have a way to go.

Is it me, or is it him?

I'm at the sink, water gushing. Ken is relaxing in the easy chair, a couple of metres away. He's begun speaking but I miss the first several words. I turn the tap off, stop what I'm doing. 'Pardon, what did you say?'

It's a common occurrence in our household. We start again, and he is annoyed.

I've had my hearing aids checked and adjusted. I understand (though Ken isn't keen to accept) that hearing aids are not a perfect solution; they can't replicate the hearing of a 16-year-old. Then there is ageing when our auditory processing ability deteriorates. It's not unusual for me to miss the first few words when someone addresses me unexpectedly; I need time to reorient myself to the direction of the sound, the pitch of the person's voice, sometimes even their accent. But with Ken, who usually speaks clearly and is nearby, it is a different matter. That is, unless other sounds are in competition, like water, the handheld Dyson vacuum or the radio, which must be turned off. It all interrupts the natural flow of conversation between two people. That's me, mea culpa, maybe.

Then there are the times when Ken and I are in conversation about, say, national politics. We might pause for a couple of minutes, then Ken resumes. But he has jumped to another topic, and I am lost. Perhaps it's still politics, but I can't immediately pick up the connection. In the pause, he's been thinking, and when I challenge him about how he got there, he takes two minutes to explain the logical steps that led him right to it. He'll accept that that's him, maybe.

Ken has had two brain operations in the past two years. His GP calls these 'a brutal assault'. Surgery, in such a delicate area, is indeed a blunt instrument, and the way the brain operates, it isn't easy to pinpoint one area and say 'that's responsible for that, precisely'. I would swear that, at times, Ken is not articulating clearly the first few words of a sentence, even if I have got the water gushing into the sink. He won't countenance that for a moment because he feels it undermines his understanding of his own reality. And I have learned not just the wisdom of letting such things go, but also of allowing the possibility that I might be wrong.

A recent MRI reminded me that while most of my large MS lesions are on the spinal cord, I do have a scattering of 'innumerable' hyperintense lesions disseminated across different areas of my brain. These have remained largely — though not entirely — stable in number and distribution over many years.

Nonetheless, I take seriously these changes in my communication ability. It crosses my mind that over the past two years of the pandemic, I've had much less face-to-face interaction with my wider social circle. Like many other older at-risk people, I've missed opportunities of any length to speak, listen and be heard. Am I just out of practice?

I've caught myself a couple of times lately, fumbling for the right word or phrase. In truth, it happens quite often. The other day, I had to laugh at myself when I was explaining to Ken that I planned to put out the 'long-legged secateurs' for the gardener to prune our thick, spiky plants. 'Oh no!' I recovered myself. 'Long-handled, I mean!'

Incidentally, Ken tells me, they are not secateurs — they are loppers. Long-legged indeed. Well, that was me.

Everyone has a story

It came to me unexpectedly in my early 20s. The realisation that the facade of a random smiling face often hides sadness, a yearning to connect the present with a different future. That what appears on the outside is not necessarily a truthful reflection of the person. That I am not the only one to have secrets.

It was not until much, much later that the privilege of deepening friendships drew me into that world behind the smile. I learned more about the lives of others than perhaps I wanted or needed to know. I'm remembering this now, because in these pandemic times, so much around me is uncertain; people are being challenged up to and beyond their limits; fragilities are being laid bare in new and frightening ways.

There's a word that describes that youthful realisation I've described. It's *sonder*, coined by John Koenig in his *New York Times* bestseller, *The Dictionary of Obscure Sorrows*. *Sonder* can be used as a noun or a verb: 'the realisation that each random passer-by is living a life' as vivid and complex as your own — populated with their own 'ambitions, friends, routines, mistakes, worries, triumphs, and inherited craziness'. *Sonder*: everyone has a story.

Sonder draws us closer to others, entering the mindset of strangers, feeling empathy before we judge. So, too, does COVID-19: 'We are all in this together,' we are told by our politicians. Because we've experienced isolation, uncertainty and fear, we can appreciate what others are going through. Does this shared ordeal help us feel less isolated?

Speaking for myself, I'm not sure. But there's another word I've discovered recently that leads me into a place where isolation loses some of its power over me. It is the Japanese concept of *yutori*: defined as spaciousness, a kind of living with spaciousness. In an interview with Krista Tippett in *On Being*, American poet Naomi Shihab Nye explains it as leaving early enough so when you get where you're going, you'll have time to look around. Or reading a poem knowing that afterwards, you can hold it, be in the space of that poem. And it can hold you, in grace.

What is my path to spaciousness? It's pausing to absorb the view from my bedroom window as I close the blinds at dusk or savouring the ending of a film that's filled and moved me, instead of heading straight for bed. It's having enough, and a little more: time, to find the words I want in writing to someone special; encouragement, for someone doing their best under difficult circumstances; money, to meet my needs and share to make another's life easier. To have enough, and a bit more — *yutori*.

Things fall apart

When both interior lights of my elevator snapped off in mid-transit to the upper floor, I was not worried. Ken would fix it. But the problem was more complex than just blown light bulbs.

The elevator had been installed in 2015 when I was beginning to experience difficulties going up the stairs. There wasn't much choice when it came to small residential lifts back then, but this one has proven thoroughly reliable. It's been serviced regularly, although in 2020 the service technician travelled from Sydney. When handed the invoice, I was shocked at how the cost had escalated.

I was in for a bigger shock when I phoned the parent company to book a service visit the following year. 'We don't do service calls anymore,' the woman informed me brusquely. 'The lift part of our business has closed down.'

Closed down? We'd been customers for over six years, and they'd abandoned us just like that, not even an email to tell us?

'We're encouraging people to find a local technician,' the woman continued, adding sagely: 'Look on the internet.'

I asked for her supervisor. The person whose job it had been to arrange service visits told me the same story, but helpfully explained what the two most likely causes of the fault would be. She thought we may be able to fix the problem ourselves, or if not, we could try an electrician. She reassured me it was not a safety issue. The elevator still worked perfectly, except for the lights.

Ken and I manoeuvred the top off the elevator and peered into its workings, looking for the batteries and the battery charger. I persuaded him that this was not a good idea and began an internet search for someone who could repair a small residential elevator.

There were companies that specialised in servicing elevators, but their portfolios intimidated me. Among the wealth of glossy commercial advertising, I searched for the word 'residential' and 'Hunter' or 'Newcastle'. Two companies I phoned were polite but had never heard of our brand of elevator. How glad I was it was not an emergency!

Eventually, a couple of days later, I found someone local. They didn't know our brand either, but a pleasant woman consulted her manager, who spoke with one of their technicians, and they were sure they'd be able to help. 'Tuesday at 7.30 am, James will be there,' she promised.

In the meantime, I resumed a project that had been interrupted by the elevator drama — writing instructions for our solicitor to make some changes to our end-of-life documents. When I was satisfied with my work, I decided to check the solicitor's office to be sure it was open.

The receptionist who took my call was a man, not the woman who usually answered the phone. When I said who I was and asked for our solicitor B, there was a pause. 'B retired 18 months ago,' the voice said, and identified himself as a senior partner. Once again, I was shocked. True, I'd not been in touch for a couple of years, but B had always been dismissive of the idea of retirement. He was proud of his fitness and long daily runs around the harbour foreshore.

It transpired that the man I'd spoken to had taken over the business B had been part of, after a period of hiatus. He'd taken my call in his car on his way into the premises, and of course would attend to my matter. As we wrapped up the call, I wondered aloud why we'd not received an email from B telling us of his retirement and passing us over to someone else in the office. 'I can't answer that,' the solicitor replied.

These recent experiences spoke to me of how easily the normal courtesies of business life can fall apart in difficult, unusual times. I felt exposed, even vulnerable, not because I was in in any danger but because of the surprising fragility of our supports. And we are not a country at war, or in economic collapse.

The word *sonder* comes to mind again. Behind that elevator company, behind that sudden retirement lies a story. Behind my phone calls and my requests lies a story. Behind those kind people who responded to me lies a story. We are interconnected, momentarily, through my reaching out for assistance on that day.

American Buddhist nun Pema Chödrön knows about these stories-behind-the-scenes. In her bestselling book *When Things Fall Apart: Heart Advice for Difficult Times*, she writes:

> We think that the point is to pass the test or overcome the problem, but the truth is that things don't really get solved. They come together, and they fall apart. Then they come together again, and they fall apart again. It's just like that. The healing comes from letting there be room for all of this to happen: room for grief, for relief, for misery, for joy.

CHAPTER EIGHT

Acts of Possession

Nothing remarkable, yet everything was

Today, my calendar reminds me, school resumes. Newcastle is still in lockdown, like Greater Sydney and much of regional NSW and beyond. It's back to home schooling for most. The Labour Day long weekend for 2021 is over, celebrated by warm, sun-filled days but not by travel further than five kilometres from our homes. Daylight saving implemented itself; each year there are fewer clocks needing manual change as automation takes over.

One of the delicious pleasures of easing COVID-19 restrictions for us is that outdoor gatherings of five double-vaccinated people over the age of 16, not counting children, are now allowed. It's been dubbed 'the picnic rule'.

One day, Ken and I met Vino and her boys in nearby Gregson Park. I packed a thermos of espresso coffee and some date muffins, both freshly made, in my mobility scooter's carrier bag. The boys' bakery favourites purchased by Ken first thing that morning were placed with delicacy on the top and the cover tucked over them. An apple turnover for Cass, cream oozing everywhere at first bite, and a custard tart for Zeus, which he likes to cut neatly into four triangles.

There was nothing remarkable about that morning, and yet everything was. Unsettled clouds lowered overhead, and I was glad of my jacket. After we'd eaten, the boys grabbed their soccer ball and dashed off to the grassy space opposite our picnic table. Bare-armed in t-shirts, they are seldom cold.

Later, Vino jumped up and joined her sons in the game, sending Cass off-field to check out the park gardens with me. Cass had often played here as a toddler in our care, running everywhere, dwarfed by the flowers, me pretending to chase him. Seven years ago — yes, I ran. Now instinctively he matched his pace to mine, slow on my walker.

All the gardens were in flower except for the rose plantings, which were on the edge of blooming.

Cass couldn't remember what they were.

'Roses,' I told him. 'And do you know what it means if you give someone a rose?'

'No'.

'It means you love them,' I told him. He nodded as we turned the corner of the garden.

I persuaded him to smell one that was almost fully opened. He stuck his nose in for a millisecond, and declared, 'Nothing, no smell!'

No chance either of getting him to bury his nose in those silky petals just a little longer.

Back home, the boys collapsed exhausted after all their activity. Zeus, on the verge of starting secondary school, threw himself on the green lounge next to me, head on a cushion at the far end. As we all chatted, desultory now, I reached over and began to rub his back. I felt him quieten, settle, saw him close his eyes. For a boy who is never still, this was something.

After a while, I asked him what he enjoyed most about our morning.

He opened his eyes and looked at me, thinking. I was sure it would be something about food. The boys are always hungry.

'Seeing you,' he said, simply.

I thought, *so beautiful*, said nothing, just gave him a small squeeze of acknowledgement. My heart full.

I turned to Cass. His long frame was spread-eagled over the lounge chair.

'And you?' I asked.

He grinned, looked at the ceiling, thinking. Definitely, this would be about food.

'Seeing you,' he replied, pausing for effect. 'And Ken.'

'I've been defrocked!'

Two weeks earlier than usual, the pair of jacaranda trees across the street look as if they are being pushed to bloom against their will. Saturday is a 30°C day and the blossoms are pinched and small. I wonder if they will dance off the trees with such carefree abandon as they did last year.

If they are feeling petulant, then so am I. It's 18 weeks since I've had my hair cut; this lockdown I've resisted having Vino cut it and have allowed it to grow. My hair is wavy, and I've never been able to tolerate when it grows longer than my usual short trim. I've done my best to accept it as it is, but perhaps because my hair appointment is within sight, irritation is getting the better of me.

Then there's what has been dubbed my 'winter eczema'. This year is the third I've suffered from it, and the worst. I've tried every treatment on offer, and every internet strategy that made even the slightest sense. Eventually I asked for a referral to a dermatologist, but I've a three-month wait to see someone.

Ken and I are bickering more these days. We become irritated with each other easily, over the most insignificant things. His short-term memory has deteriorated further since his second craniotomy in August this year. When he asks me for the third time when we're leaving for the gym, my impatience rises. Immediately, I chastise myself.

Our house was built nearly 20 years ago; we've lived in it for almost half of those. But Ken is having quite an adjustment relinquishing his role as handyman-in-chief. It's part of his identity and sense of self-worth: he's always been able to fix most things. Now his coordination, vision and fatigue issues make using tools a challenge. To me, the answer is obvious: pay someone to do what we can't manage. But it's not so simple for the person whose role is being usurped, and I realise I am over-simplifying what this means for him.

I'd much rather 'keep up' than 'catch up', knowing exactly who to call on when needed. It takes time and effort to find reliable people to help us, and this is best not left till a crisis. I am conscious that, even as the organiser, I am encroaching on Ken's turf. Delicate negotiations are needed about each new maintenance project.

I learned more about this sensitivity when one day I began to make a rice pudding. I get the best results by cooking on the stove top rather than in the oven. I set the milk and rice to bubble gently, knowing it needed constant stirring for a period of 20 minutes. Confident it had reached a safe simmer level, I popped into the laundry to do a two- or three-minute task. Ken appeared while I was absent from my post.

'Where are you?' he cried out. 'You've got to stay on the job!'

'In the laundry,' I called back. 'It's fine; I know what I'm doing.'

I hurried back to the kitchen, where Ken was stirring.

'I've turned it right down,' he admonished. 'If you're cooking, stay at the stove. Nothing in the laundry could be that important.'

'Ken!' I was annoyed. 'I've been cooking for more than 50 years — that burner was down as low as it would go!'

I picked up the spoon and resumed stirring.

The kitchen is my domain. How would I feel if someone took over my role, not allowing me to do the simplest of tasks, perhaps because I might have an accident? How disempowered would I feel then? Our small spat over the rice pudding was a salutary lesson for me: not because I didn't know what I was doing, but because I experienced how it felt to have someone doubt that I did.

My big achievement recently was locating a handyman who is capable and turns up to work when he says he will. As Ken chatted with his replacement over the tasks for the week ahead, I had a glimmer of insight into the emotional complexity of giving up a role that helps us feel needed and valued.

By evening, after a meal that included a perfectly cooked creamy rice pudding, our mood had lightened. 'I've been defrocked!' Ken grumbled, smiling.

I decided to seek out distractions from my petty resentments, ignoring the heat, my flyaway hair and itchy skin. On Tuesday, when the library was due to reopen, I would collect the books that had been in their own special lockdown, held on reserve for me for months. On Wednesday, I would farewell a friend leaving on a much-cancelled trip to Melbourne to be with her family. By then, the jacaranda trees would be releasing lavish cascades of lavender blossoms, carpeting our tiny street.

Making things clear

The end of 2021 was looming. Days of rain, of wind, of temperatures jumping from low to high and back again, unsettled everyone. Requests arrived to do things I'd not done for years, such as radio interviews and public speaking; so, too, tidings of illnesses and sudden deaths of people I've known; and other news I'd rather not hear.

That is life these days, a telescoping of experiences into a tiny space so they feel far more intense than they would normally. Omicron, a new variant of SARS-CoV-2, the virus that causes COVID-19, was about to overtake the Delta strain, its approach heralded by speculation and commentary from people who may or may not know what they are talking about.

Around this time, my so-called winter eczema without-a-rash escalated dramatically. In addition to an itchy scalp and various patches around my body, that itch sensation became overlaid by searing pain. Stabbing, burning, intermittent, intolerable pain. The lotions and ointments prescribed by my doctor were useless; only cold packs worked, for short periods of time.

After a few days of this, I'd reached a tipping point. I couldn't endure another two weeks of waiting for my dermatologist appointment; I'd seek a second opinion. After three years of failed treatments, I was in despair. My Hamilton friend Jan had recently found a new GP who she said was the most thorough doctor she'd ever had. I made an appointment with him.

Dr R took on my issue as a challenge, a problem he was determined to solve, and fast. First, he wanted to rule out potentially 'sinister' possibilities like lymphoma and multiple myeloma where itchiness-without-a-rash was a symptom. Both happened to be in my family. I was sent for extensive blood tests and a CT scan.

When the reports returned clear, Dr R settled on an interim diagnosis of neuropathic pain or neuralgia, caused by disordered and disrupted nerves. My MS was likely the instigator, hence 'under the skin, not on the skin'. Dr R prescribed an appropriate medication, and within 24 hours all my symptoms — except my itchy scalp — had disappeared. My scalp would take longer to resolve, he told me, but already much of the heat had left it.

After a few days, I could barely remember what all the fuss was about. I went to the dermatologist for whom I'd waited three months. He was happy with the course of action taken by Dr R but found a likely squamous cell carcinoma on my face on which to conduct a biopsy. A couple of weeks later, I visited my regular doctor and told him about seeking a second opinion from Dr R. I'm not sure what he thought, but he said he was glad I'd found help.

The experience reminded me of the hazard of accepting our lot when we have a chronic condition, of just going along with things and not making a fuss. My quality of life, especially my sleep, had been quite badly affected, but I put up with things far longer than I should have. I was certainly desperate when I presented to Dr R and no doubt that spurred him into action.

Getting good medical care is an interaction between patient and doctor. If there are no obvious symptoms, our doctor relies on us to tell them clearly how our complaint is affecting us. My local history friend Robert told me how recently his wife, Coralie, had 'put her back out' rather badly and the ambulance was called. As the paramedics attended to her, they asked her to rate her pain on a scale of 1–10. 'One thousand!!' she screamed. Now that's what I call making things clear.

Saying no, staying well

I have resolved to stop listening to the news. Listening, watching, even to a lesser extent reading it. I say 'resolved' because I am not sure if I'll be able to fully implement that resolution.

It began early in 2022 with the floods, especially those affecting northern NSW, where Ken and I had lived for nearly a decade. I followed the reporting, the drama of rescue, loss and devastation, deaths by water. When it came to the recovery phase, it was too much for me. How would so many thousands of people, families, children, ever reclaim their lives? How could a town like Lismore be rebuilt safely?

Russia's invasion of Ukraine was becoming more terrible, more brazen by the day. I found it utterly unbelievable. What has happened to our world order, the shared values and wisdom of the democratic West? Is it our turn to experience another Hitler?

That feeling of powerlessness in my gut rises to my chest, then my throat. I lose my voice. I don't want to know. I can give donations but do little else. I can't place my mental state on the altar of despair, even though that's what I feel impelled to do. I don't berate myself for lacking empathy, because I'm overwhelmed by empathy. It sinks me in the slough of despond, while all around me people are enjoying going about their daily lives.

Turning off the news is one positive thing I can do to fortify myself. It feels like an expression of agency. It helps my state of mind; I can think more creatively about my own life, as well as the situation of our world. Find the snippets of positive news, marvel at courage, whether in floods or war.

I choose to not be in a state of chronic arousal, triggered by the news. I've read that it spurs the release of the stress hormone cortisol, even deregulating the immune system. I'll allow more time for thinking, for concentrating, reading deeper, more thoughtful works.

The fact-bubbles popping on the surface won't help me to understand the world in any significant way. Swiss philosopher and entrepreneur Rolf Dobelli wrote in his 2014 essay 'The art of thinking clearly: Better thinking, better decisions' that it is 'the non-stories: the slow powerful movements that develop below journalists' radar that have a transforming effect and make the difference'.

By the time Dobelli's book *Stop Reading the News: A Manifesto for a Happier, Calmer, Wiser Life* was published in 2020, he'd notched up a decade of news-abstinence. The effects of this freedom for him: less distraction, more time, less anxiety, more insights. Of course, he reads — longform journalism, in-depth books and the like. It's not easy, he agrees, but it's worth it.

Another thing Dobelli says resonates for me: he explains how a misplaced sense of duty can direct our behaviour. That's it exactly — I feel a sense of duty to keep informed, up to date. A sense of duty to flooded regions, to war-torn nations, to displaced refugees. To the whole suffering world. Dobelli would argue in counterpoint that our duty is to keep an open mind so we can concentrate on complex issues and think clearly, as well as for our mental and emotional wellbeing.

I'm not sure I can be as purist as Dobelli. But I, too, have already experienced the positive effects of keeping a distance from the drama of everyday news reporting. There's a test for me ahead though: will I be able to shield myself from consuming blow-by-blow reportage on the upcoming Federal election?

Out of the fog

It was three days since I'd placed that packet of medication as high as I could reach in the kitchen cupboard. On the first day, I had a splitting headache no analgesic could touch. On the second day, the headache had gone but I'd spent most of it on my bed, deeply fatigued. This day, I am a new woman.

When I sought out a different general practitioner, I was desperate for help with my increasingly itchy skin. At that time, I would have given anything for an answer, for relief. The benefit from the first medication he prescribed turned out to be short-lived, so he prescribed another. That seemed to make a difference but there were side effects. At first, I didn't care that the medication made me feel clumsy, slowed my already reluctant gastrointestinal functioning and gave me brain fog. I would cope! By my pre-Christmas check-up though, I was considering reducing the dose slightly. Dr R agreed, noting it would be a balancing act to get an optimum outcome: side effects versus my original symptoms.

Christmas was celebrated as planned. As the January weeks wore slowly away, Vino and her family succumbed one by one to COVID-19. They were not alone — so did thousands of others. We kept to ourselves, using Skype and the telephone to connect with family and friends whose plans to visit had been forced to change. My own state worsened.

From the moment I sat down to watch the evening news on television, the itch on my scalp awoke. The neurons fired off like the crazy jumping-jack firecrackers of my childhood. Nights were difficult to bear; I ran the air conditioning to keep cool and used corticosteroid lotion for temporary relief. Clearly, the reduced dose of medication wasn't working, and I reverted to the original higher dose. It, too, failed to quell the itch that had broken through and was now spreading once again to my neck and shoulders.

That wasn't all. As the new medication no longer held back the neuropathic itch, its side effects were getting more disabling. I found it hard to complete tasks, leaving the last bit for a return attempt. I grasped for words, finding only a void. More than once, I lunged for support from an awkward position, risking a fall.

Still, I exercised daily on my cross-trainer, tackled small projects on my computer, and continued helping my older grandson practise dictation on FaceTime. To an outside observer I was functioning normally, but I knew full well how mental acuity and command of my body were sliding away. I was not coping after all.

Medications that act on the central nervous system (like sedatives, muscle relaxants, anticholinergics and antidepressants) are often prescribed for symptoms arising from MS. But they can be a double-edged sword because the central nervous system of a person with MS is easily upset. Too much of anything — including alcohol — is a risky business.

I decided on a new strategy. I would stop my medication 'cold turkey' because the side effects were unacceptable. Increasing the dosage further was out of the question. I would manage my night flares of neuropathic itch by using cold packs sooner rather than later to pre-empt the next attack.

On the third day after stopping the medication, I felt much the same as usual. As I was making my bed, though, I noticed I was working my way around it without counterbalancing on my walker. Before going downstairs, I picked up a small mending task I'd abandoned: I found a needle already threaded and sat down. As I did so, I noticed the folder of poems I'd learned by heart but abandoned a while back. As I stitched, I repeated lines from Wordsworth's 'Tintern Abbey'. By the time the repair was finished, the lines were well on the way to re-establishing their place in my memory.

Getting breakfast in the kitchen, I walked easily from end to end without touching the counter for balance. When Ken joined me, I commented on some news I'd heard earlier: nurses and others now speaking out about the true conditions in NSW hospitals. 'There's now a whole ' — I paused, grasping for the word — '*swathe* of public sector unions — teachers, nurses, paramedics — that will mobilise against this government to support Labor at the next State election.' Just a momentary pause and I'd found the word I wanted, *swathe*. Oh, the joy of small triumphs!

Walking better, retrieving words more quickly, memorising poems again, and even my fine motor coordination making a reappearance. I feel as if I've been stumbling around in a fog, only to trip over those capabilities I value most in my everyday life. As I retrieve them and hold them close, I see their value afresh. I will be careful about letting them go in future.

A trove of friends

'**I remember you're** partial to rural and tree photography,' emails stepson Peter. 'You might like this.' I click on the photo and am suffused with the damp of early morning mist. I sense the strength of the eucalypt branches, and the rough-and-smooth contrast of peeling bark over the creamy trunk makes my fingertips tingle.

At the tree's base is an iron gate, left open deliberately or perhaps in carelessness. Heading across a cleared paddock towards forested foothills marches a post-and-rail fence, a relic of past times. The hand-cut posts are uneven, some jutting high, others cut low.

Peter is becoming a fine landscape photographer, a hobby pursued as respite from his work as a respiratory nurse and the challenges of teenage kids. Most of my contact with him has been about crises in his father's health. Our connection over his photography signals a more personal direction for our relationship.

Sporadically over the past year, I've trawled through my journals to extract snippets of interest — life changes, career milestones, family events. I'm surprised at the sheer number of people I've crossed paths with, but barely remember the part some of them played in my life.

Many of my enduring friendships have come from people I've met through work. I've changed jobs more often than the average, and later, in over 20 years of private consulting, every project gave me the chance to meet new people from a different area of health services.

Looking back over those journals, I see crisis present in so many of my friendships. Navigating challenging environments such as the HIV/AIDS epidemic bound my team together like nothing else could. Our individual strengths and weaknesses were exposed, and we had to quickly learn from our mistakes and forge ahead.

Initiating and managing change in organisations, especially where some staff are resistant, became a core role in my later consulting work. At times it felt the closest I'll ever get to abseiling! But the gift has been the friendships formed right at the edge of potential disaster.

Out there, nothing can be hidden, and trust is non-negotiable.

I find that by its very nature, in the relationship that is a deep friendship, crisis can combust. Through my journals I trace periods of misunderstanding, then estrangement, and sometimes with the passage of time, reconciliation. As Cecile Yazbek notes, 'At times, the thick can become suddenly thin. It is then that I feel a sense of loss, which stays with me for some time.' The return may be slow as trust is rebuilt, but ultimately the friendship is more honest and accepting of differences than before.

I've lived in different countries, cities and towns, making new friendships with each move. While this became more difficult as I transitioned into retirement, I've found that by following my interests, whether writing and blogging, social history or improving our neighbourhood, friendships have evolved naturally.

At this time of life, though, friendships are made based on *what you see is what you get* — it is of no consequence how many university degrees one has, or what might have been achieved in one's working life. Or even, in my case, whether

I could once walk or run. I am as I appear in front of you today.

My friend Vicki Coughlan, met in my early blogging years, understands this, commenting: 'Every friendship is built on different foundations, our present challenges of isolation adding yet another layer to this complexity.'

In recent years I have been surprised to discover a friendship blossom with someone whom I've long known, but never connected with as richly as this special relationship now allows.

And do we need to invent crises in which these late friendships can be honed and crystallised? No — because crises come built in to this late stage of life. Health issues, downsizing, grief and loss: they are all there. So are inherent gifts and blessings if we look carefully. It is in this trove that we'll find our lifetime store of friends both old and new. There, for each other.

Time, missing

'**For the first** time, we were there as adults, grown up, but together.' The year was 2000 and David, my eldest son, was reflecting on the Christmas just past. He was 24.

Since finding those words recorded in my journal, I've been thinking about how our relationships with our children change and evolve throughout our lives. And how sometimes crises accelerate and colour that change.

As a family, we'd been through a lot over the previous decade, 1990 to 2000. My first husband's illness reached breaking point for both of us; then came our separation and divorce. I was diagnosed with MS. In my journal, I wrote:

> Through all this, we hold to one another
> as each of us finds the pathway forward
> for our different lives. The children's
> father remains close and within the
> circle of family support. Christmas 1999

> feels like a watershed; we've pulled through. As parents, we've given our three children roots; now it's time for them to find their wings. And they do.

After I remarry and move north to live with Ken, David and Vino find partners and create their own families. I've sometimes wondered whether my moving away was necessary for this to happen. In any case, they flourished in the spaces created between us.

One by one, grandchildren arrived, enlivening anew the bonds that connect us. The texture of intimacy changed as the focus swung from the couples to their children. After the move from Kyogle to Ballina, I journeyed often to Sydney and Newcastle, bearing gifts to celebrate birthdays and Christmases. Entranced, I got to know these new little people who have expanded our family. I learned respect for their parents, their privacy, their decisions and life choices. They are adults now.

When Ken and I relocated to Newcastle, close to Vino's family, and later Dan, we became accustomed to this new, good way of being in a family. Of living a few kilometres apart, within easy reach; David just a couple of hours distant. Then early in 2020, COVID-19 landed, and everything changed.

There is fear of the virus, and of other people. Ken and I are both immunocompromised and in the high-risk age bracket. In between lockdowns and outbreaks, we manage brief breaks away.

We take calculated risks with the Newcastle families. Our grandsons channel their vitality for us, lend us grace. In the long gaps between seeing them, they grow lanky and lean, learn new expressions and mannerisms. They get COVID-19 — their whole family does; they miss school excursions and planned holidays. Zeus graduates from primary school and moves to secondary. In a photo Vino sends me, taken at the beach, he poses with the studied knowing of an adolescent. It's happening so fast.

I've not seen David (known as Dave), Becky and their children for nearly two years. We're not the only families separated by the need for vulnerable, immunocompromised elders to protect themselves. Yet I worry about how tenuous my relationships might become with grandchildren Sam and Grace. Without the stimulus of touch and laughter, the interplay of fun and games, I feel I'm losing them; they must be forgetting me. I send presents into a void, unsure what books or games they have, what colours suit them best.

In my next contact with Dave, I float the idea of making a short visit to see them. I feel I must reach out, take the chance, that my time is running short. His response is sobering: he is back at the office in the Sydney CBD, getting the train to work; COVID-19 is everywhere; there are infections reported each week at the children's schools. He's the adult now, cautioning me. I don't tell him that, in our health district, new cases are running at well over 2000 a day. The weight of evidence is against us, for now.

I decide that I must have more faith in my children, in the way they've been brought up, in the love we share. I'm not going to lose my Sydney grandchildren: they'll understand by emotional osmosis how important we are to one another. And even if there is a gap for a couple of years, there is always the chance of something unexpected emerging, perhaps a different kind of friendship between us in the children's teenage years.

Ken and I mull over the situation, the pros and cons. 'You've got a certain risk budget,' he says, 'and it's up to you to decide how you'll use it.'

'If I must choose,' I tell him, 'I'm drawn to the new generation of my grandchildren. They are the future.'

Usually tending to pessimism, Ken surprises me with encouragement. He makes a couple of good suggestions as to how I might get to see Grace and Sam before 2022 is out. Buoyed by our exchange, I go to my study, sit down at my desk, and begin an email to my son.

CHAPTER NINE

Better than Expected

Being there

From the third floor of the office building, he's a diminutive figure walking with deliberation along the foreshore. In the background, the massive rust-red bulk of *Brave Sailor*, a Chinese container ship, glides into port, escorted by three improbably small tugboats. I grasp the vertical handles of my rhomboid exercise machine and draw them towards me.

When my session finishes, I'll put on a mask, say my goodbyes, and take the elevator to the ground floor. As I begin to ease my way down the access ramp, I see Ken waiting in the shade near the car. The passenger door is open, the hatch ready to receive my carbon-fibre black walker, chosen for its lightness to lift. Within minutes, we're on our way home.

We've been doing this for three years. It's just a routine, yet to my mind, Ken's being there is an act of faithfulness.

My sister-in-law, Lori, tells me that when she used to do her grocery shopping in a large regional town, my brother John would sit on a bench outside the supermarket and wait for her, 'people watching'. Having lived a rather isolated life on the land, he loved observing the individuality and quirkiness of townspeople. As soon as Lori reached him with her loaded trolley, he would join her in pushing it to their HiLux. Now, bed-bound for as long as I've been attending my gym, he reminisces about those times, confused and puzzled over why he's not able to accompany his wife and help her in this small way.

From the time I was a teenager, returning home to the farm from boarding school for holidays, I'd be brought a cup of tea and a coffee biscuit in bed each morning by my father. He'd done this for Mum from the time they were married. My children's father, Dick, did the same for me. Perhaps it was something older generations just did, a routine. Or faithfulness.

Daughter Vino remembers coming out of her primary school class at the end of each school day and finding her dad sitting on the bench waiting to walk her home. I knew it was part of his daily routine to stave off the demons of his depression. To her, it was 'just Dad'.

I look at my children, middle-aged themselves now, and reflect on the value each one of them places on keeping their word, being on time, doing what they said they would. If that's been passed down through the generations, I'm glad.

In our uncertain lives, these acts of faithfulness are proof we matter to someone else. Other descriptions come to mind: conscientiousness, reliability, dependability. I see them expressed in the punctuality of my hairdresser, the daily replenishment of shelves at my local IGA, the gift from a friend who knows when my spirits need a boost.

As Ken and I move cautiously out of a month of self-seclusion. I will go back to the gym; Ken will resume his city walks. After the hour, he'll be at our car, waiting. For as long as he's able, he'll be there.

In a strange land

Outside the darkened cafe that I'd expected to be open this Easter Saturday, I wait for friend and Newcastle historian Julie Keating to arrive. We'll soon find another place nearby for our coffee and catch-up. There's only a scattering of people in the street, but here's George Kiriakidis, on his way to the essential grocery business he's run for nearly four decades. We chat about the economic times: the most difficult, he says, he can remember.

Julie joins us now, and I introduce them. No one is in a rush this day, not even George. But as he takes his leave, he sums up. 'If we're lucky,' he says, 'our lives are long. And we can be unhappy, or happy. Whatever's going on for me, I choose happiness.'

George repeats this, his mantra, as much for himself as for his listener. Optimism is vital to him.

Buoyed by his cheerfulness, we move through to the next cafe, even as waves of noise from exuberant customers rush to meet us. Intimidated by the crowds, I waver at the brink, but Julie wades in. Soon she finds a secluded table at the back, piled with used crockery.

Settling ourselves among the potted plants, we ready ourselves for a long wait to be served. It's no matter. We came to talk anyway, and eventually we'll eat and drink, too.

As Saturday dissipates, so does the traffic. There's hardly a car parked in our short street. The busy through-road nearby wakes only briefly to carry the occasional traveller to the lights at the intersection and there, pause. Can silence reverberate? As Easter Sunday descends, the quietness deepens even further.

The silence calms me, and this is exactly what I need.

The world feels a precarious place right now. So many of us are just managing to stay afloat, keep fate at bay, or maybe not. The news flowing into my inbox is mostly about health issues affecting not just people close to me, but their wider friendship circles, too. I want to hold an open and supportive space for those I care about, for those being tested.

The fragility of my own situation is not lost on me. Successive trials of different medications have left me with a propensity to infections, including *Staphylococcus aureus* (golden staph); antibiotics have been added to my mix of tablets. I've sensed myself becoming more anxious, less patient, easily stressed. I haven't liked myself much. But at long last, the neuropathic itch (or dysesthesia) that has plagued me for so long is in retreat.

Recovery in my small world is slow, but it is happening. And it helps enormously that the unrelenting rain has fled; our courtyard gardens have been restored; the holiday plans of children and grandchildren are happening exactly as arranged.

Sitting outdoors on Easter Sunday morning, I'm looking forward to some quiet reading. In my lap rests Issue 149 of *Granta*, loaned to me by son Dan. I pass the palm of my right hand over its cover, pausing to sense the raised textures of the different-coloured inks. This issue is *Europe: Strangers in the Land*. As I lean against the back of the chair and close my eyes, I offer my face to the cleansing light.

Did you see?

At the cafe near the entrance to the hospital, a socially distanced queue of blue-garbed healthcare workers waited to order their coffee, heads bent over their phones. Moving along the corridor to the imaging suite, I was puzzled. Where was everyone? A couple of young doctors passed me, chatting quietly as they walked, no rush. Had something happened?

I was at John Hunter Hospital for a routine MRI scan. The air was fresh, the corridors clear of parked equipment. I realised what was missing — visitors, and people lining up for PCR tests as when I came here in 2021.

I was early for my appointment, and the waiting radiographer whisked me off to get changed. A young man, maybe 30, he showed not the slightest sign of boredom explaining a process he must have repeated innumerable times to patients like me. Anticipating my needs, he manoeuvred my weak right leg onto the table with care.

Next, wedging a small soft-but-firm pillow on either side of my neck, he explained, 'This is to support your head, stop it from moving.' I'd not had such a pillow before, and as I wriggled into comfort, I marvelled at the feeling, as if my head was being cradled by celestial hands.

Afterwards, I had some time to fill in before being collected so I dawdled back towards the cafe. I was surprised to notice an art exhibition stretching along the walls of the long corridor — Arts for Health. And here, in this distant hospital, my suburb Hamilton appeared — all the works on display had been generated in a creative workshop space there called the Hudson Street Hum. Its name — inspired several years ago by a story on my *Hidden Hamilton* blog — celebrated the industrial community that flourished in Hudson Street in the early 1900s.

I paused to read vignettes by some of the artists, like this one from Lynnette Passeri:

> It's Friday morning and I'm at my happy
> place. For a few hours I allow myself
> to focus on only what is happening in
> the moment. Guided by our art teacher
> Peter Lankas . . . these classes have been

a godsend during these extraordinary times.

Daydreaming my way along the paintings and enjoying the serendipity of my discovery, I remembered my first meeting with Suzie and Aleeta, who had founded Hudson Street Hum. I'd been impressed by these exceptional women, as they had shown off the soaring spaces of the former warehouse they were converting. Their vision was for a social enterprise that brought artists, writers and makers together to learn, create and communicate, paving the way for similar initiatives in Hamilton.

Later, I take my coffee outside the hospital to the pick-up and drop-off zone, finding an entire bench free in the shade. I sit down and remove my mask; the air feels lively, almost vibrating. Waiting for my transport in the clear afternoon light, coffee in hand, is a simple act. Allowing myself to know this, I am happy.

Rushing in

It's easy to panic when our circumstances change suddenly, especially as we age. It's the feeling that our lives are suddenly accelerating in a particular direction, and we are powerless to interrupt the trajectory.

Our future housing needs preoccupy many of us in the later stages of our lives. Some older people are looking to downsize, others for a better location or even just a change. It's a challenge to get the timing right. Several friends toy with the idea of downsizing, and some, like me, have partners with worrying health conditions. We could find ourselves alone at any time.

A widow I know, whom I will call Vera, panicked when she had a couple of bad falls and felt her memory was deteriorating. She was living in a beachside suburb of Newcastle, enjoying an active community life, especially with her church. She sold the family home and bought a smaller one near her daughter in one of the outer suburbs.

Once there, however, she began to feel isolated and trapped; it was difficult to forge new friendships at this late stage of her life and her daughter and family were busy with their own lives. Realising she'd made a mistake, Vera purchased a villa in an over-55s complex in our street. Reconnecting with her old friends and interests just 10 minutes drive away, she enjoyed four or five happy years before being admitted to an aged care facility.

Occasionally Ken and I discuss how I might manage in our present house if I was alone. It is well located, close to shops and services, and has been adapted to my mobility issues. But like any house, it needs upkeep and maintenance.

A year or so ago after one of Ken's melanoma scares, I panicked. I insisted we look at a small house for sale in Vino's suburb. We didn't inspect it, just drove by. It was cute but squashed in among other houses. Vino was away at the time and on her return, we told her about it.

'Mum!' she exclaimed. 'Don't sell your house! I'm only 10 minutes away. How could you ever be better off anywhere else?'

Since then, at regular intervals Ken reminds Vino, 'When I die, don't let your mother rush into selling the house!'

I've thought about having a university student to board with me, possibly an international one. I could offer a large bedroom, a walk-in wardrobe and ensuite bathroom. I'd trade accommodation for a few hours of help each week. I'd enjoy having a young person coming and going.

The housing crisis is acute for women approaching the end of their working lives, without sufficient superannuation. Another option might be a woman in her late 50s, early 60s, perhaps still working, who would be interested in a similar trade?

That said, I could also imagine myself living alone in a ground floor villa, just two bedrooms and a small garden. It's good to think about the future and test out various scenarios. I have friends who are in housing situations in which they are at some risk; they will need to move eventually, but, because they are coping for the time being, prefer to delay for as long as possible.

In deciding the timing of a move, we are managing risk. This calls for a clear-eyed weighing of the facts of our individual situation. We may not get it perfectly right, but nearly right is probably fine. While we remain cognitively and emotionally able to do this, we are safe.

Nevertheless, it is important to be prepared. Moving in a crisis can be a real panic situation and that's when we make poor decisions. If a move must be made suddenly, someone else will have to sort out our lifetime's accumulation of possessions. I want to do my own sorting, while I still can.

It does help to have younger people in one's circle. People who are fit and able and willing to help, especially in an emergency. It may be sons or daughters, friends, neighbours or people we employ. But we are an ageing cohort, so time and capacity to do this for each other is running out.

Reading the tea leaves

'**We got it!** We got it!' Two voices in unison and two beaming faces appeared out of the lift at our gym.

'The house you were looking at earlier in week?' I asked, already knowing the answer would be, 'Yes!'

I'd come to know two sisters — Marion and Anna — as we each worked on our machines, exchanging snippets of information about our lives in between deep breaths. I'd learned that not only did they live close to each other, they lived in the same street. It had been a deliberate decision a few years back to co-locate in Newcastle where they'd grown up, Marion moving from Sydney and Anna from the Gold Coast.

I'd assumed they'd each lost their husbands, but our conversation hadn't dug that deep. Having been thinking and writing about the housing decisions that face us as we age, I was impressed by what they'd done.

Things changed when Anna had a stroke. Tall and reed-slender, she was shocked to find herself in John Hunter Hospital for weeks, followed by outpatient rehabilitation. Joining our gym was a natural next step for her. She works out assiduously and one would never guess there was residual damage. But the event forced the sisters to think again about their living arrangements:

they got on well; what was the point of maintaining separate houses and large gardens?

The search for a house began. They had no fixed views about which suburb, but were adamant the house should suit their individual lifestyles, with plenty of space. They found what they were looking for. One of their houses had already been sold so they were able to snap this one up immediately.

Our gym class of nine, plus our exercise physiologist, had followed the house search with vicarious interest. That morning, we all shared the sisters' delight with their perfect find. They were due to settle the purchase within a month and would be in their new house before Christmas.

Marion and Anna had already made one important decision and it had paid off. In relocating close to each other in Newcastle, they had confirmed they would be happy to create a new home together in their old hometown.

So here are two capable women approaching 70, unafraid of change, who know what they want and are fit and well enough to make it happen. They have 'read the tea leaves', acknowledging that health risks lie ahead — especially for Anna

— and acting to minimise those risks by moving in together. Luckily, they are best friends and have each other: it's a solution unique to them and wouldn't suit everyone. But it's a timely example of a pivotal life decision that will, hopefully, prove to be a good one.

Forgotten taste

A headline caught my eye in *The Sydney Morning Herald*. 'The forgotten taste of uninhibited joy: Yemenis win over Saudis.' A football match, Yemen's under-15 boys soccer team won the West Asia junior football championship. A wave of ecstatic pride swept a country riven by civil war, where millions are displaced and, in the words of a United Nations spokesperson, are 'marching towards starvation'.

For just a brief time, people spilled into streets to celebrate these boys who'd lived half their young lives surrounded by wartime violence. Revelling in the forgotten taste of uninhibited joy brought much-needed relief from the daily hardships of life under siege.

I reflect on how we as humans have the capacity for joy in the midst of suffering — in itself a cause for celebration. As is the fact we can gather *en masse*, shoulder to shoulder, social beings that we are, singing, dancing and calling out, oblivious to the press of bodies around us.

My own situation pales into insignificance in comparison with what happened in Yemen. But as Christmas 2021 approached, I had the smallest taste of what it was like to be surrounded by friendly, joyful faces, everyone in a celebratory mood.

The occasion was the 150th birthday of my suburb, Hamilton. The local association of business owners had organised a feast of activities as a 'coming out' from COVID-19: performances, art activities, dancing and music, food carts and Santa appearances. Colourful and engaging, the celebrations carried on from morning to night, drawing crowds from all over our city.

I was asked to be involved because of my local history research and writing about Hamilton, much of which is now evident in the streets. Blue-and-white heritage plaques on buildings, mosaics and etchings in the pavement and art installations in the re-envisioned plaza tell the story of this 19th-century coalmining settlement. A heritage walk I'd designed in 2016 had been digitised for a mobile phone app and the City of Newcastle had asked me to speak at the launch.

In the lead-up to the celebration, I gave radio and print media interviews, then a speech on the day. None of it was easy for me. I was several years older than when I'd last done something similar, promotion for my books. This time, preparing for these activities felt like getting ready for an arduous examination. On the day itself, I spoke to the outdoor crowd from a seated position on my walker, which was not ideal. But afterwards the rewards were great, as I reconnected with people who have enthusiastically contributed to my Hamilton work.

There were photos to be taken of course. In one group photo, Santa lent his arm to help me keep my balance at his side. Councillor Carol Duncan manoeuvred my walker out of the way and returned it to me after the shot, which was taken by her husband. In more ways than one, it felt like a family affair.

When the group photo was posted on social media, I emailed it to Dave in Sydney. 'Mum,' he wrote, 'it's so good to see you doing something light-hearted!'

Dave's remark made me realise how much of these past two years had been a hard slog. Keeping safe, caring for my family, trying to stay well myself. Like the people of Yemen, joy had almost become a forgotten taste. Certainly, the bursting, uninhibited experiences of joy had been elusive in the extreme. Little did I realise then that this would be the last time for many weeks that I would feel free to move among people without fear of COVID-19.

Yet I know I can still savour the experiences that steal upon me unexpectedly and reveal themselves to be so much more than I'd thought. In his poem 'From Blossoms', Indonesian-born American poet Li-Young Lee writes about buying peaches from a boy at a roadside stall, holding them in a paper bag:

> O, to take what we love inside
> to carry within us an orchard, to eat
> not only the skin, but the shade,

not only the sugar, but the days, to hold
the fruit in our hands, adore it, then
   bite into
the round jubilance of peach.

CHAPTER TEN

In Focus

Perfect pledge

Christmas Eve, 2003. Ken and I had a private marriage ceremony in the Kyogle Court House. It was a second marriage for both of us.

The first thing that stands out from my blurring memory of that event was finding a witness. On our arrival, Kim, the Court Registrar, welcomed us warmly. Her assistant would be one witness and she'd promised to find another on the day. That proved harder than she'd thought on this busy Christmas Eve.

It was Ken who jumped up from his chair and dashed into the street, after Kim had made several fruitless phone calls. He accosted a young First Nations Bundjalung woman who was just getting out of a car and persuaded her to be our second witness. Wearing jeans and a snug-fitting red singlet top, she had the lithe grace of a runner. Curls cascaded down her back, their blackness seared by a few faded auburn streaks.

Following Ken, her dark eyes were liquid with amusement.

As they swept back into the foyer, there was a small cheer of triumph from we three waiting women. Amid introductions and laughter, our small group moved into a nearby room.

I remember our wedding vows.

With the witnesses, Ken and I stood in front of Kim. Formal now, but with the edges of her mouth still fluid with smiles, Kim gathered her papers and spoke to them.

> 'We are here today to witness the
> marriage of Ruth and Ken, and to
> wish them every happiness in their life
> together . . .'

I fixed my eyes on Kim's face and forced myself to listen to her measured voice. Emotions jostled on the edge of my awareness; mentally, I barricaded them. Kim's words stepped through.

> 'The primary basis of their relationship
> is dialogue and openness, a willingness
> to share oneself with the other, to
> expose oneself and one's needs and

> concerns, and to accept the other self and their needs and concerns. To love is, above all, to act for the sake of the other, to act for the good of the one to be loved.'

I had read these words in our preparation phase; back then I'd been impressed by their modernity. Now, in this plain functional room, the words leaped out at me as if afire — *expose oneself, accept the other self, act for the sake of the other, for the good of the one to be loved*. Trembling, I reached for Ken's hand. It was warm, alive and totally enclosing. He'd agreed to take me as his lawful wedded wife. Now it was my turn.

'I will,' I said firmly.

Almost two decades later, I've been married to Ken longer than my first marriage. It's been different from what I'd expected, but as Ken grapples with a terminal health condition, those vows seem more significant than ever. If I'd searched for months before our marriage, I could not have found more moving and appropriate vows. From that modest country Court House, the Registrar produced the perfect pledge.

What a high calling, to act for the sake of the other, to act for the good of the one to be loved. What an honour to be the recipient of that action; equally to be the giver. I want to fulfil that vow, right to the end. It is my commitment, my gift, to my husband.

More than a sign

'I'm exhausted,' sighs Ken, crumpling into the easy chair, laying his head back and closing his eyes. 'Utterly exhausted.'

It's 9.15 am. He's driven me to the gym on the harbour foreshore, walked 4000 steps, and shopped for four items at the Woolworths Metro. This new, cut-down version of a Woolworths supermarket doesn't overwhelm Ken. The shopping list is short so he can memorise it; we rehearse briefly before setting off in our separate directions from the car. It's a chance to pick up sourdough bread warm from the oven, fresh fruit or something a bit different from the chiller section for dinner.

Once home, I make coffee on our machine. I feel virtuous, having been up and active early. From the third-floor gym, I've absorbed the sights and sounds of the wakening port, noted the motionless billows of steam suspended above the Orica chemical plant to the north and smiled at the sight of white cockatoos taking turns to swing crazily on the halyard of our building's flagpole. People of all ages exercise with vigour and intent, along the riverside path. I never fail to feel invigorated, these two mornings each week.

For Ken, though, there is no wind to lift his sails. Now beginning a seventh month of immunotherapy for the melanoma metastasis in a lymph node in his groin, he's been stalled by side effects. He's receiving just one drug this time, nivolumab, which reminds immune cells to attack cancer cells anywhere they can be found. While the side effects he's experienced so far aren't life-threatening, they can make daily life a struggle for him.

For many weeks now, stiffness and an awkward gait have troubled him, especially in the first half of the day. His weak right side and hip are culprits. I've noticed his responses and reflexes are much slower than before; his short-term memory is affected. Underpinning everything is fatigue.

Nothing we can't manage, but Ken feels and knows he is not his usual self.

A recent PET scan has thrown some light on his hip problem. There's inflammation in the synovial fluid of the surrounding capsule: a recognised but rare adverse event of nivolumab. I worry that it might morph into an autoimmune disease like rheumatoid arthritis, but Ken's oncologist puts these fears to rest. Anti-inflammatory medications are prescribed. He counsels Ken to focus on the big picture, that in these past six months, no additional metastases have appeared. The existing one has grown a fraction but seems under control. We are grateful.

Ken has joined a melanoma support group on Facebook and is finding out first-hand the best and worst of social media. Seeking facts and figures, he finds mainly emotions. He is incredulous at the tidal wave of responses received by a woman asking for advice on how she can arrange her hair to best disguise the scar from her craniotomy. Yet he has had some useful interactions and acknowledges Facebook's power in bringing together people who otherwise would never connect. Like the rest of us, he is learning to use it in a way that works for him.

Every three months, Ken has surveillance scans to see how his cancer may be changing. There's a brain MRI and a PET scan of the body. The word *scanxiety* has been coined in the cancer community to capture the feelings that people experience around this time. Imaging appointments and blood tests must be arranged and attended; then comes the wait to visit the oncologist and hear the results. Afterwards, if the news is good, there's a huge sense of relief. A reprieve: life can resume. The alternative is another matter.

A travel program on Italy, presented for television by British actor Richard E. Grant, provides a welcome distraction. Naples, resting in the shadow of the volcano Mount Vesuvius, was one of the cities featured. I learned that, three times a year, a special mass is held in the city's Cathedral of the Assumption of Mary in honour of the patron saint of Naples, San Gennaro (Saint Januarius). What is believed to be his bones and blood are preserved as relics in the cathedral.

During mass, the presiding Archbishop opens a safe containing a reliquary with a circular sealed vial filled, it is said, with the saint's dried blood.

What happens next is of critical importance as to how the people of Naples will live their lives in the months ahead.

A miracle is believed to have occurred if the dry, red-coloured substance on one side of the vial becomes liquid, covering the entire glass, when the reliquary is moved from side to side. Disaster is averted. If the blood fails to liquefy, calamity is signified — war, famine, disease, even an eruption of Vesuvius. When the blood does liquefy, however, it is as if the people are set free in a miraculous way.

Despite my scepticism about the miracle, the power of the event for those gathered in the great cathedral was undeniable. Joyful exhilaration swept the crowds as they left, confident in the sign they'd just received from their supreme saint.

I connect this with how it feels in our home every three months when Ken receives his results after a couple of weeks of *scanxiety*. This week good news for him isn't a saint's blood liquefying: it's *nothing happening, no new activity, nothing to see here.* It's the product of high-powered technology that can scan a person's body and miraculously, detect where disease may be on the move. Or not.

It's more than a sign, it's information.

Yet like the fire smouldering deep within Vesuvius, the scanning process still contains some mystery. Radiologists can interpret the scans with all possible skill and care; we can consult the runes and the relics for signs of hope and favour. Still, what is unknown remains out there, beyond sight and sense. In the end, I conclude, it is our ability to go on living day by day with an element of mystery that holds us strong.

Pieces of a puzzle

It appeared as if by magic, with a proprietorial air as if it had always been there in my neighbour's backyard. Neat and almost elegant, its V-shaped roofline matched the house, and the tops of two French doors peeped invitingly above the fence.

A week or so earlier, nearby residents had been letterboxed with a notice to say our street would be closed for some hours around midnight. Then a crane would airlift the pre-built studio over the fence, to settle on the concrete slab prepared for its arrival.

My neighbour is a sculptor, and she's been planning this for well over a year, maybe more. She wants to work from home, and to see more of her teenage son. Our street is abuzz; everyone approves. There's more work to be done, integrating it into her backyard with decking, pergola, steps and so on. But the studio is the core structure.

Something else surprising occurred in my own life that week. Not solid and tangible like the studio, but an insight that, for me, was just as substantial.

I was visited by a staff member from myHomecare, the aged care provider that supplies Ken and me with 'domestic assistance' — two hours of cleaning once a fortnight. She was to do an annual review; this was my first.

Karina Coutts was warm and professional, and during the hour and a half, she completed various forms on my behalf and even gave me some advice on how to improve the shine on the glass walls of the shower recess. I assured her I was very happy with the person who cleaned for us; he was hardworking and dependable. Some of Karina's questions about my health issues and functioning were quite probing, but her discretion and obvious knowledge of client needs reassured me. I assumed the funding body had to know that the help I received was justified.

After a while, when I was beginning to think this interrogation would never end, she asked me what goals I would like to set for the coming year.

Goals? I wondered. Skirting boards dusted more often? Clean under the stove and behind the refrigerator? She could see I was flummoxed.

'Well,' she offered, 'the first one could be your physical strength. You've told me about the gym you attend twice a week, and how every year the exercise physiologists measure changes in your upper and lower body strength. One goal could be to continue to improve, so you don't have a fall. And keep doing the housekeeping you clearly do already, that's not covered by our program.'

'Oh,' I replied. 'That's good, I get what you mean.'

'Can you think of another?' she pressed gently.

'We've spoken about the meal delivery program I've started,' I suggested. 'It's with another provider, not yours. I'm so pleased to have found excellent meals at last, especially spicy vegetarian ones! The goal is to relieve me of at least some of the burden of cooking dinners every night, and always having fresh meat and vegetables in stock. There's less risk of me having an accident related to cooking hot meals, plus we're getting a more varied diet.'

'Excellent,' Karina replied, typing fast. 'Can you think of one more?'

'Gardening,' I replied, getting the hang of this now. 'Over the past two years, since Ken has become less able to do physical things, I've been working with various helpers to simplify our courtyard gardens. I aimed to get things to the point where I can take care of them myself — without tripping over the hose or having a fall moving pots around. I have a gardener now, private, not under the aged care program. My goal is to be able to maintain the gardens with her help and be safe.'

'That's great!' enthused Karina, finishing her typing. 'Each of those goals contributes to your overall objective of remaining in your home as long as possible, adapting to changes in your own and your husband's lives.' So that's how she's linked it all back to my fortnightly clean!

Happy with her morning's work, Karina drove off to interview one more client before lunch. The aged care service was very fortunate, I reflected, to have someone of her calibre. She'd achieved what all good interviewers seek to do: through their questioning, to open space for the person being interviewed to see things differently, and to have new insights.

I realised that like my neighbour with her art studio, I now have structures in place to underpin my continuing independence. Through Karina's interview, I could see how all the pieces of the puzzle fitted together, forming part of a bigger picture. There are no guarantees of course, but readjustments have been made in our living arrangements to give Ken and me a decent chance of managing well for some time yet.

The insight had appeared magically, like the studio, but doesn't belie the large amount of planning that goes into setting such structures in place. Most of it is the result of my own initiative and determination. I've decided that I, too, can be pleased with my endeavours.

If things become urgent ...

It had been on my 'to do' list for months — contact two or three local aged care homes and ask for a tour of their premises. I'm familiar with such facilities, but I've never actually been inside one in Newcastle since moving here nearly a decade ago.

Like most people my age, the prospect of this as my final home fills me with dread and provokes an immediate, fierce denial. The report of the Royal Commission into Aged Care presented to Federal Parliament in February 2021 confirmed my every fear.

Ken and I have discussed the possibility of either or both of us needing residential care, though he is adamant it won't be him — he thinks palliative care will most likely be his end-of-life pathway.

'Anyway, you've got eight years to go before you need to start worrying,' Ken asserts. 'For women, the average age of permanent entry to residential aged care is 85; for men it's 82.'

I argue that because of my MS, I'm not average — in fact, I've got a substantial handicap.

One of my legs, indeed the whole of my right side, is already compromised. Anything that takes out my 'good side', even temporarily, is bad news. In the past, I've had glimpses of what it might be like when severe sciatic nerve pain strikes there. I could be in a wheelchair, needing someone to help me with my personal care. This would be beyond Ken in his current state, and how long I could manage with home care would depend on the severity of my injury and/or disability.

Ken quotes more statistics: the average age of entry to a home care program is 81 for women, and 80 for men. 'That proves my point!' I declared. 'I got my first home care assistance when I was 74!'

I allowed this task to languish at the bottom of the list, until news from a friend in a distant city spurred me into action. One night, her partner collapsed in the bathroom. My friend was unable to move him, the ambulance was called and her partner was admitted to hospital. It soon became clear he was not expected to come home. He would be needing high-level residential care for the rest of his life. My friend's shock and distress were upsetting in the extreme, and my own dormant fears and insecurities were triggered.

I'd developed a short list of three aged care facilities to check out. The first one (Anglican) set in lovely gardens is the most expensive. Although it has expansive Merewether views, it is a little out of the way for prospective visitors. I've learned quite a bit about it, as my hairdresser's grandmother is a resident there.

The second one (Baptist) is more centrally located in Waratah, a few blocks from where my son lives and a short drive from my daughter's place. It, too, has pleasant gardens and the rooms (called suites) have been recently renovated. Its CEO is innovative and a strong public advocate for the sector.

The third facility on my list (Uniting) is in my suburb, Hamilton. It prides itself on being 'like home', the staff and residents an extended family.

It also claims a groundbreaking 'household living' model, so while a resident has their own bedroom, they share kitchen, dining and living spaces much like the home they've left. My 92-year-old neighbour thinks she'll move there eventually.

Despite my children declaring they won't allow me to go to a nursing home, things are not so simple. I've always liked to research my options, and to be prepared.

Any expectations that I'd be scheduling visits to each of these facilities in the coming weeks were dashed as responses came back. Yes, they do arrange tours for two people at a time, but none at present because of the COVID-19 lockdown. So — 'keep in touch, and in the meantime, please fill in this application form'.

The forms presented by each aged care home are the those required for seeking immediate admission. I've explained I'm 'planning for the future, checking out options', but the forms are still necessary. I comply and wait. At least I'm having a practice run at the forms, which are a challenge even to a person with all their faculties.

After the forms are submitted, it is as if I've become a member of a club. I've demonstrated my *bona fides*; nothing is too much trouble. One email concluded: 'And if things become urgent in the meantime, please call and I'll see what we have available.'

I feel a little shaken by the whole experience, as if I've had an encounter with a night stalker. I've drawn close to that which I've long feared. I'm 'on the books', and I have an offer if things become urgent. Perhaps that's enough for now.

Secret life of EBV

'**The cause of** multiple sclerosis is unknown; there is no cure.' This pronouncement accompanied the diagnosis I received in 1997.

While there is still no cure for this mysterious autoimmune disease, there are now excellent disease-modifying therapies. And on 13 January 2022, research findings were published in the journal *Science* confirming what has long been suspected, a compelling link between the Epstein-Barr virus (EBV) and MS.

A member of the herpes family, EBV is one of the most common human viruses. It eventually infects about 95 per cent of adults, but very few will develop MS. EBV is best known as the virus that causes glandular fever, an acute viral infection called infectious mononucleosis affecting mainly young adults. While it may not necessarily cause symptoms, EBV can remain latent in cells and may sometimes reactivate.

The study to test the hypothesis of a link between EBV and MS was huge — more than 10 million active-duty US military personnel were studied between 1993 and 2013. Researchers from the Harvard T.H. Chan School of Public Health calculated that people infected with EBV were 32 times more likely to develop MS than people who had not been infected with the virus.

This strong association between EBV and MS risk suggests that EBV is part of a chain of events that leads to most cases of MS. The researchers are not yet claiming causality. Although it is known that the SARS-CoV-2 virus causes the disease COVID-19, and the human immunodeficiency virus (HIV) causes AIDS, the cause of MS is multi-factorial.

EBV alone is not sufficient to trigger MS — other unknown factors play a role. For instance, about 200 genes have been identified that each contribute a small amount to the risk of developing MS. Environmental factors such as how far people live from the equator, smoking, childhood and adolescent obesity (especially in girls), and low vitamin D levels are among the factors implicated.

I contracted glandular fever as a young adult — I was 23 — and became extremely ill. I was a Residential Tutor at St Ann's College at The University of Adelaide, while teaching English at The Methodist Ladies' College. I learned that I'd been delirious and hallucinating, with a high fever. Anxious friends and a doctor were at my bedside for hours, days.

It was a challenging time of my life when I made decisions that I later regretted. Despite the severity of my illness and the stress of life circumstances, I recovered well. Yet, as we now know, EBV had become ensconced in my cells, to await the confluence of conditions perfect for it to reactivate.

The Harvard researchers don't yet understand the specifics of the part played by EBV in initiating MS, in concert with other unknown factors. They seem confident, though, that if a vaccine was available to stop EBV infection, most cases of MS could be prevented. In retrospect, I was one of the unlucky ones, infection with EBV significantly increasing my risk of MS.

When something happens to us, like being struck down by an incurable disease whose cause is not known, it is natural to ask, 'Why me? What was there in my constitution, my genetic makeup, or my lifestyle that predisposed me to develop this condition?' I've not been particularly intent on finding the answers to these questions, but I remain curious. For years, as suspicions about EBV grew, I wondered whether there might have been a connection between my illness in Adelaide as a young woman, and MS diagnosed almost 35 years later.

Does knowing part of the answer help?

A little, but I've long since accepted that what's done is done. There will be no sliding doors moment to enable me to make different decisions that could have altered the trajectory of my life. Cecile Yazbek commented on my blog:

We are a distillation of years of work,
growth, the cultivation of insight and
so much more. Time and how we spent
it has enabled us to see through things,
to find the value, to question ourselves,
and finally to settle into this time now.

That seems a fruitful place to be.

Leavings of our lives

The big plastic storage box was empty, all my Hamilton local history research papers finally disposed of. Some found homes with fellow local history writers; most were binned; one last bundle of survivors was filed in a binder labelled 'Working on this'.

I doubt I'll ever do more 'working on this'. Naming that binder was creating a last resting place for papers I couldn't bear to throw out. As

I skimmed their contents, dithering over a decision about their proper fate, I wondered what other people do with such troves. I've distilled the best of knowledge and stories from them into my *Hidden Hamilton* blog and two published books. But there is still ever-more interesting information, unused.

The fact is, so many of the possessions collected in our lifetimes are of interest and use only to ourselves. They will be a burden if left to someone else to decide what should go in the waiting rubbish skip and what to keep. I've long since disposed of the body of work and supporting papers from my health consulting business. This Hamilton endeavour was the hobby of my retirement years and is the last to go.

Over the past week, I've said goodbye with thoughtfulness and respect.

The documents I agonised over longest were handwritten letters. There is an abundance of emails and comments made on the Hidden Hamilton Facebook page and elsewhere in cyberspace, but these are out of sight and out of mind. Every print media article about a new stage of my work stimulated fresh correspondence — mainly from older people, those who collected the local papers from their newsagent and wrote with pens on blue lined writing pads.

Some wrote simply to thank me and share their delight at finding stories about the suburb they loved. Rob happens to be internet savvy, but his opening was typical:

'I've just discovered your blog about Hamilton. I couldn't stop reading it once I'd started. I have lived in Hamilton all my life and have no desire to live anywhere else. I can't tell you how much I loved growing up here.'

Rob grew up in the Gatekeeper's Cottage with a bomb shelter in the front yard and a well in the back. He'd collect coal thrown from passing steam trains slowing to negotiate the curve, taking it home to his grateful mother. Rob helped me identify the long-lost location of the Station Master's house, now grassed, and planted with scattered trees.

Others wrote to tell me their stories, their family histories, some lengthy. One man warned me he was going to bore me! He didn't, and we became friends.

What were the writers expecting me to do with their outpourings? I always replied or telephoned if they gave me their number. When

I was able to draw new information from these accounts, I added it to the relevant blog post. But mostly I felt overwhelmed and inadequate to the task of responding. Was it enough, I pondered, that something I'd written had triggered their memories, providing a reason for them to set pen to paper, and connect with someone who cared?

I realise that for the average person, the leavings of our lives can't be captured and preserved to endure beyond our memories or our lifetimes. Seated amid a slew of papers, I find myself really wanting to do that but knowing it to be impossible. My books will go out of print soon; the day will come when I'll be unable to maintain the functionality of the blog as a reference for the occasional searcher.

What comfort then can I glean from this last remaining box of papers? I know that some of my correspondents have passed away. Julie Lomax's joy was beyond bounds when in 2016 I told her that the 1940s black-and-white photograph of her father outside his fruit shop had been chosen for the cover of *More Hidden Hamilton: Further Stories of People, Place and Community*. And even more ecstatic when she saw the finished product: the stacked produce arrayed behind her dad transformed into luscious juiciness by publisher Christine Bruderlin's subtle colouring.

Sometime after Julie died, her daughter found my name in her mother's address book. She phoned me to tell me the news, and to say what an inestimable gift I'd given her mother in her last years. Job done, I think; job more than done.

Good things come ...

How do people change over two years? Do older people change more than younger ones? I waited with anticipation to see 'my Sydney family', from whom I'd been separated by the pandemic, Ken's and my vulnerability, unpredictable and relentless rain, and the everyday busy-ness of a growing family.

Rain threatened to derail this visit, too. All week I checked and rechecked the weather radar and forecasts, noting every subtle change. Dave, Becky and their children, Sam and Grace, were coming for the weekend. The first event of their visit was to be a family lunch at In Forno, an appealing Italian restaurant in my suburb with indoor seating and outdoor tables under an atrium abundant with hanging plants.

Late in the week, I dropped by to discuss our table selection with owner Harry, a rising entrepreneur. To him, I was entrusting my hopes for a lunch that would be successful in every possible way. 'Don't worry, Ruth,' he assured me. 'The weather on Saturday will be fine. I know!'

I stopped worrying. After all, Harry would be studying the vagaries of the weather with the utmost dedication because the day-to-day organisation of his business depended on it.

When Dave and his family appeared at our front gate, I was slightly bemused — they hadn't changed at all! Yes, the kids were two years older, but they were mainly taller and familiar to me from FaceTime. Dave and Becky seemed to have mellowed into middle age, softer at the edges, relaxed. They'd not become strangers after all. What little faith I'd had!

Harry was true to his word. Not only did the rain stay away, but the food he provided and the setting he'd arranged delighted us all. I've not laughed so much — since the pandemic began. Indeed, good things do come to those who wait.

After lunch, while Becky, Vino and I gossiped over our coffee, Dave disappeared with the four young cousins. He returned later with a noisy, ecstatic bunch, jumping up and down and brandishing their loot. They'd been to Jim's, a milk bar and lolly shop remembered from past visits and spied on the walk to In Forno. Despite all the pizza they'd eaten at lunch, they still had room for something more. 'It's a separate compartment in our stomachs!' Zeus explained to me later, his grey eyes mischievous.

My lifelong friend Leigh says that sometimes she thinks of our lives as tidal. The 1990s of which I've written in the micro-essay 'A tumultuous decade' were a high tide mark for her, too. A time when water comes in at the flood, bringing nutrients and rejuvenation to the many forms of life left stranded by the low tide. A time of change and new beginnings.

This day, it's not a decade I look back on as a high tide point in my life. It's simply a weekend, connecting with loved ones I'd not seen for too long, gathering my dispersed family to celebrate being together.

Tidal energy, I've read, is renewable because at its source, it is never depleted. It is power produced by the surge of ocean waters during the rise and fall of tides.

The joyousness of that brief weekend will supply me with all the energy I need for the bleak winter months ahead. Would it be foolish to hope that, like the wind, the sun and the tides, the energy of joy, too, is renewable?

Are we there yet?

Spring was in sight, and I'd made what I thought would be the last big pot of soup from barley and winter vegetables. Then a sudden cold front swept through NSW, turning the Blue Mountains white under a cloak of snow. The Great Western Highway and other roads were closed; high parts of NSW shivered under minus-zero temperatures. On the coast we suffered gale force winds and shivered, too.

Despite this, positive signs are mounting. Overarching them all is a new Federal Government making thoughtful commonsense decisions, reminding Australians that it is possible to feel proud of their leaders.

COVID-19 graphs are heading down. Experts agree that the wave of deaths and hospitalisations has peaked but they are divided on the question of deaths. Ken and I have escaped COVID-19 so far and have not had any of the lesser respiratory infections. We've just received our fifth dose of the vaccine. I still wear a mask when I leave the house.

Australia has come though the BA.4 and BA.5 subvariants of Omicron, but is it over? No epidemiologist is brave enough to answer yes or predict what might happen next. On the balance of probabilities, they say, another variant or subvariant is in the wings, and may well appear in the months ahead, before Christmas.

Over the winter, my dysesthesia has been mildly reactivated. Pre-emptive use of a cold pack on my neck and scalp helps, and I am confident that if the itch worsens, the necessary medications are to hand. My health and wellbeing have been better than for many months.

Ken has completed nine months of immunotherapy, undertaking regular hospital visits for infusions. This treatment could go on for at least another year if no new tumours appear. He's learned from his Facebook melanoma support group that even if he stopped treatment now, there is no guarantee the side effects he's been experiencing would disappear. Most insidious is fatigue — one member reported still experiencing it seven years after ceasing treatment. For us, there's no relaxing our guard while the coronavirus ponders its next mutation.

When I began the *Morning Pages* blog in 2020, I was preparing for the worst. By the time Ken emerged from his second craniotomy, I expected he might live for months, not years. I didn't consider how long I'd write for, except that *Morning Pages* would probably end with Ken's death. Two years have passed, he is still here and reasonably well. Now, as I bring this book to its close in mid-2022, it is time to pause and reflect on where this journey has brought me.

The past two years have revealed what living with the uncertainty of cancer feels like. It's not all that different from what I've been doing for 25 years with MS, with one great exception. For

Ken, early death is the issue; for me it is disability exacerbated by age.

I've always sought to learn as much as possible about MS, take control of my treatments and lifestyle, and, importantly, get on with life. It was my great good fortune to be well enough to work until my late 60s. In Ken I have a partner who has been proactive in planning our finances so that our present and future care options are assured, as far as possible. I feel for those without such security, as financial challenges added to disability or ill health can limit choices and increase hardship immeasurably.

Ken struggles with accepting the uncertainty of his health situation and longs to feel like the person he once was. He's not there yet. That's his journey, and as we pledged nearly 20 years ago, we will continue to act for the good of each other for as long as we live.

And what of joy, where my writings began?

Joy bloomed for me when I entered MacLean's Booksellers, Hamilton's tiny independent bookshop, to choose a book for grandson Zeus's birthday. Each time I visit, I feel embraced and calmed, immediately at home. In an alcove at the far end, I pored over offerings found for me by a young staff member who seemed to have road-tested every children's book in the shop. Before long, she had placed the perfect one for Zeus in my hands.

I felt joy, with a dash of pride, when Cass telephoned me to rearrange our speech coaching session on FaceTime. 'I have to go to the dentist,' he explained, 'but what about five o'clock?' His voice was clear and resonant, every sound crisp, his careful sentences whole. Is he there yet? No, he has further to go. But after that telephone call, I have released my fears for his future. Like a flock of rosellas startled from the grassland on which they are feeding, they rise, swerve and disappear into the blue. The boy will thrive.

Over these past two years I've chafed at finding my life constrained, feeling I was losing engagement with the wider world and missing the variety I'd once enjoyed. But during the pandemic, I learned to focus on what was close to me, discerning beauty and care in small moments and simple interactions. Experiences of my daily life, no matter how insignificant, took on a singular shape and intensity.

As I recorded what I saw, heard and felt, a more mindful way of being and thinking unfolded. Was it possible that while my life had slowed down, it had not shrunk after all? Through these processes of mindful attentiveness, could it have deepened — expanded, even — into the smaller spaces that are my waking hours?

Am I there yet? Like my walking, or not walking, it doesn't matter. While I've mourned my losses, I've realised that my life need not be defined by what I am unable to do, but by what I can. And I have discovered *yutori* — that exquisite Japanese concept of spaciousness mentioned in my micro-essay 'Everyone has a story'. Living with spaciousness, I arrive early and have time to look around, to see something I would not have noticed if I'd been rushing. I have enough of everything for every day — and a little more. *Yutori.*

Acknowledgements

My thanks go to everyone who appears in this book, named, renamed or unnamed. Wherever you live, you are the fabric of my life.

I wish to gratefully acknowledge permission granted by writers Melanie Cheng, Pema Chödrön, Josie George, Antjie Krog, Li-Young Lee, Alex Miller and Marge Saiser to quote previously published material. Details of their publishers and works are in the addendum, Permissions.

Thank you to the followers of my *Morning Pages* blog, for reflecting on my musings and sharing your thoughts. Your comments on my posts reassured me that my writing would resonate with a wider readership.

Thank you to editor Shelley Kenigsberg, whose perceptive eye and light touch gave me confidence in what I have written. Designer Christine Bruderlin, thank you for mentoring me through the book production process with your customary skill, insight and care.

Finally, special thanks to my husband, Ken, for being part of my story — and continuing, so far, to defy the odds.

Permissions

Grateful acknowledgement is made to the following for permission to quote previously published material:

© Cheng, Melanie, 2019, *Room for a Stranger*. Published by The Text Publishing Company, Australia.

> Three things he could feel. Three things he could hear. He could feel the pillow beneath his head, the wooden bedframe in his hand, his hair resting on his forehead. He could hear a motorbike storming past the house, the distant cry of a child, birds chirping outside the window. He concentrated on his breathing.

Chödrön, Pema, 2016, *When Things Fall Apart: Heart Advice for Difficult Times.* Shambhala Publications, USA.

> We think that the point is to pass the test or overcome the problem, but the truth is that things don't really get solved. They come together, and they fall apart. Then they come together again, and they fall apart again. It's just like that. The healing comes from letting there be room for all of this to happen: room for grief, for relief, for misery, for joy.

George, Josie, 2022, Founder of the blog *Bimblings* at https://www.bimblings.co.uk.

> What a surprise it is: I have slowed down and I did not drown. My life is imperfect, hard, uncertain, but it is here, it is happening in my body and my body is alive, and to notice it again feels like baptism. Outside, the world races ahead and leaves me behind, but for the first time in a long time, I don't think I mind.

Krog, Antjie, 2009, *A Change of Tongue*. Penguin Random House South Africa.

> But nowadays this larger world is incessantly present in your yard and on your stoep (verandah) and in your guest room and in your kitchen, it takes up so many seats at the table, it always has a whole mouthful to say about your food. Because of television and newspapers, you are now saddled with this other world. And you want to get rid of this other world, you wonder desperately how you are going to overcome it. *Intimacy with your own world* is the one thing that enables you to survive this ever-present other world.

'To Hold' from 'Behind my Eyes' by Li-Young Lee. Copyright © 2008 by Li-Young Lee. Used by permission of W.W. Norton & Company, Inc.

> So often, fear has led me
> to abandon what I know I must relinquish
> in time. But for the moment,
> I'll listen to her dream,
> and she to mine, our mutual hearing
>   calling

more and more detail into the light
of a joint and fragile keeping.

Li-Young Lee, excerpt from 'From Blossoms' from *Rose*. Copyright © 1986 by Li-Young Lee. Reprinted with the permission of The Permissions Company, LLC on behalf of BOA Editions, Ltd., boaeditions.org

O, to take what we love inside
to carry within us an orchard, to eat
not only the skin, but the shade,
not only the sugar, but the days, to hold
the fruit in our hands, adore it, then
   bite into
the round jubilance of peach.

Miller, Alex, 2017, *The Passage of Love*. Allen & Unwin, Australia.

Not knowing what we have to say and
having nothing to say are not the same
thing. We find out what we have to say
when we attempt to say it. We think we
want to say one thing, then in the attempt
to say it we find there is a deeper and
clearer truth waiting for us just below the
surface of our first thought.

Saiser, Marge, 2019, from 'I Save my Love' in *Learning to swim.* Stephen F. Austin State University Press, USA.

> I save my love for what is close,
> for the dog's eyes, the depths of brown
> when I take a wet cloth to them
> to wash his face. I save my love
> for the smell of coffee at The Mill,
> the roasted near-burn of it, especially
> the remnant that stays later
> in the fibers of my coat.

Bibliography

Al-Majahed, A. and O'Grady, S., 'The forgotten taste of uninhibited joy: Yemenis win over Saudis', *The Sydney Morning Herald*, September 15 2021.

Cameron, Julia, *The Artist's Way: A Spiritual Path to Higher Creativity*, Pan Books, London, 1993.

Cavafy, C. P. (K. P. Kavafis). The poem 'Ithaca' was written in 1911. During his lifetime, the Greek poet, journalist and civil servant Cavafy refused to formally publish his work, preferring to share it through local magazines and newspapers. His most important poems were published two years after his death, which occurred in 1933. The translator for the excerpt used here was Rae Dalven, and the poem can be found at *https://ninaalvarez.net/2007/05/03/poem-of-the-day-49*

Cheng, Melanie, *Room for a Stranger*, Text Publishing, Melbourne, 2019.

Chödrön, Pema, *When Things Fall Apart: Heart Advice for Difficult Times*, Shambhala Publications, Boulder, Colorado, 2016.

Crews, James, *Every Waking Moment*, Lynx House Press, Amherst, MA, 2021.

de Botton, Alain, *Status Anxiety*, Hamish Hamilton, London, 2004.

Dobelli, Rolf, *Stop Reading the News: A Manifesto for a Happier, Calmer, Wiser Life*, Sceptre, London, 2020.

Fry, Kathryn, *The Earth Will Outshine Us*, Ginninderra Press, Port Adelaide, 2021.

George, Josie. Founder of the blog *Bimblings* at https://www.bimblings.co.uk Author of *A Still Life: A Memoir*, Bloomsbury Publishing, London, 2021.

Krog, Antjie, *A Change of Tongue*, Penguin Random House South Africa, 2009.

Lee, Li-Young. The poem 'From Blossoms' in James Crews, ed., *How to Love the World: Poems of Gratitude and Hope*, Storey Publishing, North Adams, MA, 2021.

Lindbergh, Anne Morrow, *Gift from the Sea*, Hogarth Press, London, 1985.

Miller, Alex, *The Simplest Words: A Storyteller's Journey*, Allen & Unwin, Crows Nest, 2016.

Miller, Alex, *The Passage of Love*, Allen & Unwin, Crows Nest, 2017.

Nye, Naomi Shihab, interviewed by Krista Tippett in *On Being* at *https://onbeing.org/programs/naomi-shihab-nye-before-you-know-kindness-as-the-deepest-thing-inside*

Saiser, Marge, The poem 'I Save my Love' in *Learning to Swim,* Stephen F. Austin State University Press, Texas, 2019.

Shedd, John A., *Salt from My Attic*, The Mosher Press, Portland, Maine, 1928.

Tallerico, Brian, writing for the film review website *RogerEbert.com*, 2021.

Vertosick, Frank Jr., *When the Air Hits Your Brain: Tales of Neurosurgery*. W.W. Norton & Company, New York, 2008.

Wagner, Jenny, *John Brown, Rose and the Midnight Cat*, Penguin Books Australia, 1980.

Yeats, W.B., 'The Lake Isle of Innisfree', *National Observer*, UK, 1890.

About Ruth Cotton

Ruth Cotton grew up on a sheep and cattle property in the north-west of New South Wales. After qualifying as a secondary school teacher at the University of New England in Armidale, she set off to explore her interest in other cultures. This led her to work in Fiji and, later, Malaysia. Back in Australia, Ruth began a career in the public sector, in spheres as varied as international cooperation, Aboriginal education, and health. In the late 1980s, she played a key role in the NSW response to the HIV/AIDS epidemic. For the last 20 years of her working life, while living with multiple sclerosis, Ruth ran an influential consultancy business, facilitating change within Australian health services. Since retiring, she has blogged and written on the local history of her suburb, her family's history and daily life with multiple sclerosis. Ruth has three children and four grandchildren, and lives with her husband in Newcastle, NSW, Australia.

Stay in touch

🔗 ruthcotton.com.au
📷 @ruthmareecotton

www.ingramcontent.com/pod-product-compliance
Lightning Source LLC
Chambersburg PA
CBHW020315010526
44107CB00054B/1851